PENGUIN ANANDA

AYURVEDA ADVANTAGE

Vicram Sharma is director and a third-generation stakeholder at the family-owned Shree Baidyanath Ayurved Bhawan, India's century-old brand of Ayurveda remedies and supplements with an enduring legacy. He attended the prestigious Doon School in Dehradun and is an alumnus of the London School of Economics and Political Science. He has an intimate, practical knowledge of Ayurveda and has some of India's most renowned *vaid*s on speed dial. Vicram spent his growing years learning immersively at Baidyanath's production units across the country, where medicines were prepared using traditional methods and the purest ingredients. He is a passionate advocate for environmental sustainability and animal rights. Vicram is a hands-on father to an energetic four-year-old.

Celebrating 35 Years of
Penguin Random House India

AYURVEDA ADVANTAGE

An ancient science for modern living

Vicram Sharma

PENGUIN
ANANDA

An imprint of Penguin Random House

PENGUIN ANANDA

USA | Canada | UK | Ireland | Australia
New Zealand | India | South Africa | China | Singapore

Penguin Ananda is part of the Penguin Random House group of companies
whose addresses can be found at global.penguinrandomhouse.com

Published by Penguin Random House India Pvt. Ltd
4th Floor, Capital Tower 1, MG Road,
Gurugram 122 002, Haryana, India

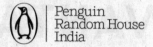

Penguin
Random House
India

First published in Penguin Ananda by Penguin Random House India 2023

ISBN 9780143455301

Typeset in Adobe Garamond Pro by Manipal Technologies Limited, Manipal
Printed at Replika Press Pvt. Ltd, India

www.penguin.co.in

MIX
Paper from
responsible sources
FSC® C016779

In remembrance of my grandfather
Pandit Ram Dayal Joshi and my grand-uncle
Vaid Pandit Ram Narayan Sharma,
the founders of Baidyanath.
My deepest gratitude.

Contents

Preface

I am my parents' firstborn. When I was an infant, my grandmother would tie a little bundle of neem twigs and turmeric roots to the carved wooden post of my crib to keep away mites and negative energies and to cleanse the surrounding atmosphere. You could say I imbibed Ayurveda from the day I was born, and perhaps even earlier, for my mother was cared for throughout her pregnancy using all the traditional Ayurvedic therapies and remedies of the Baidyanath household.

And so it is only fitting that this book, too, was conceived at the time of the birth of my own firstborn. My mother and I had moved to Anand in Gujarat for the baby's arrival. Shortly after we moved there, the country went into a total lockdown in March 2020 due to the Covid pandemic. Isolated from the outside world, we spent hours chatting and enjoying each other's company. It was then, perhaps for the first time that I realized the depth and breadth of her knowledge of Ayurveda. I had known that she had trained under the eminent *vaid*s Pandit Ram Raksh Pathak[1] and Pandit Brihaspatpati Dev Triguna[2] soon after she had married into the Baidyanath family, and later under Baidyanath's own expert in-house vaids, Vaid Sukhram Babu, Pandit Vishwanath Sharma and Vaid Deo Nandan Tripathi, but it was only then that I had an insight into her masterly grasp of the subject.

The timing was auspicious and serendipitous, for in the rough and tumble that is the hallmark of modern living, it is rare to find a hiatus long enough to allow you to engage intensely with a person or a subject. But this was a once-in-a-lifetime moment when the whole world had hit the pause button. It was a time to reconnect, look within and take stock. When the world struggled in vain to grapple with a strange virus whose origin, treatment and spread remained unknown as it marched inexorably across continents, my thoughts returned again and again to Ayurveda, the science of life—a science so complex and subtle that it made modern medicine look almost rudimentary. A science that went far beyond the nuts and bolts of biology and chemistry to address human health in the context of the individual psyche and universal consciousness. A science that bridged not only all other life sciences but was also the bridge to the cosmic.

My mother had a natural, instinctive understanding of the science of Ayurveda, easily criss-crossing the physical and non-physical aspects of health. So I asked her to teach me. What followed were months of intensive learning as she poured out her knowledge to me, as a guru to a *shishya*. Day after day, I questioned her on the basics of Ayurveda and we discussed the subject. I took copious notes and sometimes made recordings on my phone as she spoke. As I received transcripts of these recordings, I began to compile and organize these fascinating interactions, fleshing out the bare bones of something that had until then been only a sketchy idea in my mind.

Over the past years, I had seen many of my friends, especially those who had hit their forties, spend vast sums of money on products and cosmetic procedures that promised youth and beauty. These ranged from exotic Korean potions to non-surgical as well as surgical interventions. At such times, I would remember my feisty grandmother and grand-aunts, who, even when they were well into their eighties, had a clear, glowing complexion and glossy hair. Their teeth were intact, their bones strong, their energy levels high and their mental faculties as sharp as someone half their age. They never used allopathic medicines, treating themselves instead with supplements and remedies from the Baidyanath pharmacopoeia. My mother herself is an exemplar of Ayurveda's power of immunity. Despite being particularly vulnerable due to her age, as well as being a kidney donor and a cancer survivor, she sailed unscathed through the pandemic. This despite air travel and frequent exposure. She has always been a regular user of Ayurveda's immunity-boosting tonics.

Though I was the director of one of India's legacy Ayurvedic pharma companies, I was aware that there was much that I needed to learn about this complex and fascinating science. Even though I had grown up in and around the Baidyanath factories, running around as a boy among barrels of medicaments and cauldrons of simmering potions, I had not really undertaken any formal study of the subject. To correct this gap, I scoured the bookshops of Delhi looking for user- and beginner-friendly books on Ayurveda. I was disappointed to find that most books available on the subject were overly technical, dry and impenetrable. I made up my mind that this was a situation I needed to correct. I decided to write a book on 'everyday Ayurveda', one that would make this precious knowledge accessible to the layperson. But like many good intentions, this one too was put on ice as I became more and more caught up in the business side of Baidyanath—until the opportunity presented itself fortuitously and auspiciously when my son was born.

During this period of forced isolation, I sent for textbooks from the Baidyanath archives, immersing myself in the subject. On my return to Delhi, I also consulted with our family vaid, Ashok Kumar Singh. Greatly enthused by the project, Vaidji offered invaluable insights, helping me build and shape the material into a coherent narrative. One of the outfalls of the Covid-19 pandemic has been a renaissance of Ayurveda, yoga and other holistic paths to health. The pandemic has brought home to us the limitations of modern medicine and there has been an upsurge of interest in alternative healing systems. The time is right for a handbook on the Ayurveda 'advantage'.

A special thanks to Bharati Motwani for her guidance.

As this book goes into print, my son Shivay is nearly four years old. It is my wish and blessing that this book shines the light on Ayurveda across the world, and that my son upholds the torch lit by his great-grandfathers, the founders of Baidyanath.

1

Approaching Ayurveda

'Ayurveda is the most sacred science of life, beneficial to humans both in this world and the world beyond.'

—Acharya Charaka

Ayurveda is an exciting discovery of the true self that you are. And we warmly invite the reader to take this journey with us into the sublimely mysterious secrets of our body, mind and soul using the vehicle of Ayurveda.

According to sacred literature, Ayurveda originated from Brahma, one of the Hindu triumvirate deities of Brahma, Vishnu and Mahesh. He is supposed to have passed on this treasure to his son Daksha Prajapati. It is said that Daksha taught it to the Ashwini Kumaras, the twin Vedic gods. One of the earliest treatises on Ayurveda, the *Charaka Samhita*, attributes the origins of Ayurveda to Atreya. Another early treatise, the *Sushruta Samhita*, claims that the science was first propagated by Dhanvantri, who is today worshipped as the patron deity of Ayurveda.

Ayurveda is a vast and deep science of the 'body-mind-soul' bonding. It is also an effective tool to upgrade the quality of our daily lives.

Ayurveda is a holistic and multidimensional approach to living a healthy and balanced life. A careful study reveals that it is a finely structured science based on a sophisticated understanding of human physiology and psychology. Ayurveda emphasizes the integrated, holistic nature of life.

What is wellness but a serenely balanced state of mind and body aligned perfectly with the spirit that dwells within? If we address only the body, there is much that we miss. While Ayurveda certainly has a vast array of methods to heal specific bodily issues, it is so much more. It is a deep resource that teaches us that every cell has a pulsating cosmos within it. It leads us to a unique way of living—from the body, through the mind, into the spirit.

Before we address the problems of the body, Ayurveda directs us to look at our lifestyles.

Do we move our bodies enough?

What kind of thoughts do we feed our minds?

What are our dietary choices?

Are we at peace with our professional choices?

Are our relationships harmonious?

We need to regularly monitor the above to uphold the innate strength and capabilities gifted to us at birth.

Many diseases are merely outward expressions exposing the inward poverty of our minds and the negativity of our thoughts. It is unwise to attempt quick fixes that suppress bodily symptoms of diseases without holistically healing the 'being' behind it all. A quick fix is almost always temporary in nature and it is only a matter of time before the problem resurfaces or remanifests itself in some other way. It is time to cast aside this imbalanced way of living. Fortunately, Ayurveda shows us how to reclaim the dignity of health and helps us ascend to higher levels of wellness.

The Sankhya philosophy suggests that we understand our origins in order to understand ourselves. According to our revered scriptures, consciousness first existed in an unmanifest state in the cosmos. From this universal consciousness emanated soundless vibrations that led to the manifestation of Aum, which sages believe is the pulse of the universe.

Sankhya, in which the science of Ayurveda is rooted, is one of India's six famous systems of philosophy. Sankhya posits that in the beginning was choiceless awareness. This supreme intelligence, present everywhere, is referred to as Purusha, the male principle. It is complete and whole in itself, encompassing all that is pure. Hence, it is also called Atman or Satya. Upon this eternal field of pure existence there awakens the divine feminine potential, which is pure energy and creative will, and thus a womb to all desires. This is Prakruti. Thus, upon Purusha, the primordial force field, Prakruti enacts her 'creative will'. The universe is born out of the union of Purusha and Prakriti.

Since consciousness is non-material, how shall we understand the presence of matter? Ayurveda says there are two basic principles that explain the nature of reality—the principles of 'being' and 'existence'. 'Being' is Purusha, the indwelling supreme witness that is 'egoless pure consciousness'. It is formless, beyond time and space and even beyond cause and effect. Prakruti is the 'force in motion' that attains form

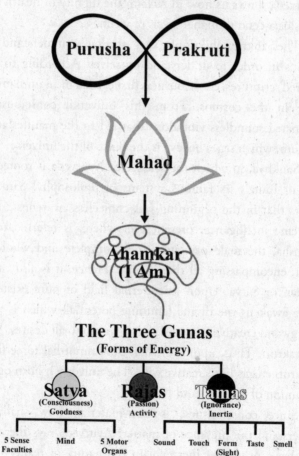

Sankhya Philosophy
(Creation & Evolution)

Purusha   Prakruti

Mahad

Ahamkar
(I Am)

The Three Gunas
(Forms of Energy)

Satva
(Consciousness)
Goodness

Rajas
(Passion)
Activity

Tamas
(Ignorance)
Inertia

| 5 Sense Faculties | Mind | 5 Motor Organs | Sound | Touch | Form (Sight) | Taste | Smell |

and has an intense desire to multiply. From the interplay of Purusha and Prakruti, the worldly mind and body spring forth from the time-space continuum.

Each of us represents a microcosm of Purusha and Prakruti. Everything in the cosmos—indeed, the very cosmos itself—is born of the union of these two. Here, it is important to keep in mind that both Purusha and Prakruti are one. One does not exist without the other. These two principles are worshipped in India in the form of Shiva and Shakti, where Shiva is pure consciousness and Shakti, its creative force.

From the union of these all-encompassing twin forces is born *mahad*, which is better understood as cosmic intelligence. Mahad is the very seed of what is and governs nature's laws. In each of us, mahad exists in the form of innate existential intelligence, as *buddhi* or intellect and as our perception of what is real and unreal. Mahad is best understood as the 'orderly cellular intelligence' in each cell of our bodies. The transmission of intelligence between cells is referred to as prana, the life force. The interaction of buddhi or the intellect with material form gives birth to *ahamkar*—ego or the sense of differentiated self.

Within this individuality, Ayurveda postulates three components or qualities, known as the *gunas*, which form the existential fabric of life. These are *satva, rajas* and *tamas*. The first quality, satva, imparts the characteristic of pure awareness. The second quality, rajas, lends the individual the dynamic qualities of motion and action. The third quality, tamas, refers to organic matter that causes inertia and a lack of consciousness.

In Ayurveda, it is important to understand the presence of the elements of the *panchtatvas* or *panchmahabhutas* in our bodies as well as in all existence. These are the subtle vibrating living forms of the five elements: ether, air, fire, water and earth. As these five elements of the cosmic consciousness are present in us, man is a microcosm of the cosmos itself. Thus, we arrive where we began—each individual is part of the whole. Without a proper understanding of these origins of human physiology, we cannot diagnose our bodily issues or diseases. This is how Ayurveda's wisdom will help us get back to a lifestyle that is wholesome, holistic and even sacred.

Unravelling Our DNA

Noted Ayurvedic physician Vasant Lad enumerates the genetic constituents of the sperm and ova. These relate to the twenty-three pairs of chromosomes that are present in every human being.

Atman, the soul or conscious principle
Manas, the mind
Agni, the metabolic fire
Soma or bliss
The five elements of ether, air, fire, water and earth
The three doshas of *vata, pitta* and *kapha*
Ojas, tejas and prana
Each of the twenty gunas in ten pairs of opposites, such as heavy and light, cold and hot, oily and dry etc.

2

Decoding the Fundamentals

At the core of all life sciences is Ayurveda. It is a holistic and multidimensional approach to living in a healthy and balanced manner. Ayurveda is based on medicine, philosophy and spirituality.

The three gunas

Satva (*satoguna*), rajas (*rajoguna*) and tamas (*tamoguna*) form the base of all human existence. They manifest as the mind, the five sense faculties, the five motor organs and the five basic elements (panchtatvas).

These three gunas can be said to have attributes synonymous with those of the divine trinity.

Brahma → Satva → Force of creation

Vishnu → Rajas → Force of vitality/motion of the organic
and inorganic in the universe, pure kinetic energy
Mahesh → Tamas → Force of destruction

The five elements (panchtatva)

In the human body, as in the cosmos, the three gunas
manifest as panchtatva or the five basic elements of ether, air,
fire, water and earth. Each of these five elements is present in
every human form and every other living form.

Ether or *akash* is that dimension from which everything
is manifested and into which everything returns. It is best
understood as that cosmic field in which events occur. Akash
has no physical existence.

Air or *vayu* has no form. It is matter in the form of gas. Its
attribute is motion, movement and mobility.

Fire or agni is that element which converts substances
from solid to liquid to gas and vice versa. It has no substance.
Its attribute is that of transformation.

Water or *jal* is matter in its liquid form. Jal has no stability
and is always in a state of flux.

Earth or *prithvi* is matter in its solid state. The attributes
of prithvi are stability, rigidity and rootedness.

There is a direct relationship between the five elements
and our senses. Ether is related to hearing, air is related to
touch, fire is related to vision, water is related to taste and
earth is related to smell.

In the human body, the five elements or panchtatva
manifest as the *tridosha*—the three biological energies of vata,
pitta and kapha.

Each one of us has all the tridosha manifested in our bodies. Every individual is born with a particular tridosha configuration, which can also be described as their constitution. This remains more or less constant throughout their life. The proportion and combination of the tridosha vary in every person. All the functions of the body, mind and consciousness are governed by the tridosha. The tridosha doctrine is Ayurveda's unique treasure and has unparalleled potential for healing in a revolutionary manner. The balance of the tridosha in the individual human constitution is the nucleus of Ayurveda.

Doshas: the big trinity of vata, pitta, kapha

'Dosha, dhatu, mala, mulam hi shariram'—Sushruta Samhita

('Our bodies are the sum of our doshas, tissues and waste.')

The panchtatva originate from the all-pervasive cosmic energy that creates all life. In the human body, the panchtatva is present in the form of three basic biological energies of vata, pitta and kapha, i.e., the three *doshas*. The term dosha comes from the *Charaka Samhita*, the oldest and most authoritative canonical text on Ayurveda, and also from the *Sushruta Samhita* and the *Ashtanga Hridaya*. The three doshas manifest in an individual as the subtle presence of the five elements and are responsible for holding together the human form. Further, through the web of our DNA, they formulate the blueprint of our dynamic physiology.

Binding our body into a form, the doshas run the bodily functions in a balanced way. It is the doshas that are responsible for the movement of the nutrient fluids back and forth and also for lubricating and maintaining our cellular structure. The three doshas are present everywhere and in every cell as its natural protective phenomenon, and yet are always in a state of flux.

Vata is formed from the elements of ether and air. It is the air element present in our bodies. It is important to understand that the air in our body is different from the air in the atmosphere. Vata means 'that which moves', best understood as the air principle in our system. Vata governs our breathing and directs all biological movements.

Pitta is formed from the elements of fire and water. It denotes fire, though this not to be understood literally—it is the heat energy in our body. It governs our body temperature, absorption, digestion, assimilation, metabolism, intelligence and perception.

Kapha is formed from the elements of earth and water. It refers to the biological water in our body. It provides the material required for our body structure. It governs our physical resistance, hydrates the skin, lubricates the joints, provides energy in the form of strength and stability, helps memory retention in the brain, heals wounds and supports the maintenance of the immunity of the organs.

It is very important to understand that vata, pitta and kapha are subtle forces that are acting upon the physical substances of our body. Ayurveda emphasizes that in order to live a harmonious and balanced life, we need an effective combination of the functions of our body, mind and consciousness. Vata, pitta and kapha collectively ensure this. Kapha governs anabolic changes, which simply means that kapha turns simpler molecules into complex ones that store energy. Pitta governs our metabolic changes, which are the synthesis of proteins, fats and carbohydrates, which form the tissues to store energy. Vata governs catabolic changes, meaning that it breaks down complex molecules to form simpler ones. The first two (kapha and pitta) help to store energy, while vata breaks down and releases energy via catabolism.

Ayurveda defines seven types of constitutions based on the tridosha:

1. Vata
2. Pitta
3. Kapha
4. Vata pitta
5. Pitta kapha
6. Vata kapha
7. Vata pitta kapha

There is no definite or conclusive method to define a person's constitution. Though the basic constitution is fixed at birth, the doshas tend to be in a state of flux. Due to this variability, an individual's constitution too can fluctuate at different times.

'Any disturbance in the equilibrium of dhatus (tridosha, body tissues and waste products) is known as disease. The state of their equilibrium is health.'—Charaka

The following are indicators that can provide a general understanding of one's constitution.

Table 1: Body type indicators

	Vata body type	Pitta body type	Kapha body type
Physical appearance	Physique and muscles poorly developed	Physique and muscles moderately developed	Physique large and heavy, stocky, inclined towards obesity
	Difficulty in putting on weight, bones and veins prominent	Moderate weight	Heavy weight
	Shoulders small, thin, at times hunched	Shoulders medium in size	Shoulders broad and thick
	Scanty hair	Moderate hair, inclined to excessive hair fall and early greying	Abundant and thick hair
	Skin dry and rough	Skin soft and warm, easily develops bruises, acne, rashes and sunburn	Skin smooth, soft and moist
Activity	Overactive, fast, restless, erratic	Purposeful, focused, forceful	Easy-going, steady, relaxed

	Vata body type	Pitta body type	Kapha body type
Mental and emotional makeup	Indecisive, nervous, anxious and worried under stress	Critical, decisive, irritable, throws tantrums, angry bordering on furious	Bold, stable, patient, unfazed, going silent under stress
Resistance and disease	Weak resistance to disease, weak immune system. Prone to pain, arthritis, problems of the nervous system	Moderate resistance to disease. Prone to infection, fevers and anxiety	Good resistance to disease. Prone to congestive disorders, asthma, inflammation, oedema
Sleep	Light, inclined towards insomnia	Moderate but good in quality. Wakes up easily	Heavy, deep. Wakes up slowly and with difficulty. Snores loudly
Sexual tendency	Erratic and variable. Strong desire but low on sexual stamina	Passionate and dominating. Moderate sexual stamina	Quite constant sexual desire. Good sexual stamina

The seven dhatus

Dhatus are the constructing tissues of our body. The seven dhatus are:

1. *Rasa* or plasma
2. *Rakta* or blood

3. *Mamsa* or muscle
4. *Meda* or fat
5. *Asthi* or bone
6. *Majja* or bone marrow and nerve tissue
7. *Shukra* or reproductive tissue

After digestion, the nutrition present in the essence of the consumed food is converted into plasma, which in turn supplies nourishment to the other dhatus in the following order: plasma to blood to muscle to fat to bone to marrow and nerve tissues to reproductive tissues.

In Ayurveda, the vital life energy is referred to as prana. Every human is a *prani* and once prana exits the body, the prani is no more. Everything that has life has prana. *Pranic* energy is like a current that circulates through the blood, passing through the entire body and powering the motor organs and sensory functions. It is responsible for respiration, circulation and intelligence and for kindling agni within the body. According to Ayurveda, all living forms have pranic energy. Prana has five variations based on its functions.

The five pranas

1. **Prana**, whose seat is the brain and which governs the intelligence, sensory and motor functions, especially those of the nervous and respiratory systems.
2. **Vyana**, whose seat is the heart and which governs circulation, joints and muscle movements.
3. **Samana**, whose seat is the small intestine and which governs the digestive system.

4. **Udana**, whose seat is the throat and which governs energy, speech, memory, will and inhalation-exhalation.

5. **Apana**, whose seat is the lower abdomen and which governs the maintenance of semen, the development of the foetus, the excretion of faeces, urine and menstrual fluids.

Koshas and Chakras

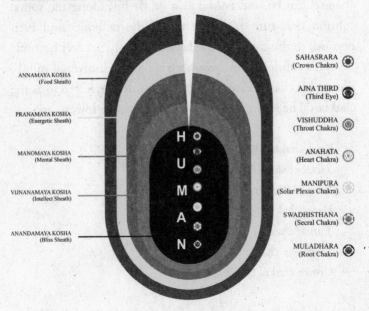

ANNAMAYA KOSHA
(Food Sheath)

PRANAMAYA KOSHA
(Energetic Sheath)

MANOMAYA KOSHA
(Mental Sheath)

VIJNANAMAYA KOSHA
(Intellect Sheath)

ANANDAMAYA KOSHA
(Bliss Sheath)

SAHASRARA
(Crown Chakra)

AJNA THIRD
(Third Eye)

VISHUDDHA
(Throat Chakra)

ANAHATA
(Heart Chakra)

MANIPURA
(Solar Plexus Chakra)

SWADHISTHANA
(Secral Chakra)

MULADHARA
(Root Chakra)

Universal Consciousness

The *koshas* refer to sheaths or layers of the atman or self. Koshas are like the many layers of an onion. The atman has five distinct koshas: the *annamaya* kosha (sheath of food), *pranamaya* kosha (sheath of prana/energy), *manomaya* kosha (sheath of thought/mind), *vijnanamaya* kosha (sheath of intellect/wisdom) and *anandmaya* kosha (sheath of bliss).

The outer life events of our body and the material world form our objective experience. The experiences of our mind form our subjective experience. Different dimensions and vibrations of experiences, thoughts and emotions form images and are linked directly to the mind and kosha connection, which further gives rise to one's perception. The mind operates within these koshas via a central channel. The channel can be understood as a subtle line along the spinal column that runs from the tip of the tailbone, and even beyond, to the crown of the head and up to 3.5 feet beyond.

This subtle channel connects us to the 'universal mind'. Along this channel are seven energy centres, referred to as the chakras. The seven chakras, starting from the lowest, are:

Root chakra (*Muladhara*)
Sacral chakra (*Swadhisthana*)
Solar plexus chakra (*Manipura*)
Heart chakra (*Anahata*)
Throat chakra (*Vishuddha*)
Third eye chakra (*Ajna*)
Crown chakra (*Sahasrara*)

Each chakra is connected to a particular kosha. The chakra system is related to the autonomic nervous system, which in turn is connected to the brain. The brain works in tandem with the five koshas, which in turn work in tandem with the seven chakras, thereby feeding information to every cell of the body. Thus, the mind, koshas and chakras form the very axis of the mind–body complex.

3

Agni: The Fire of Life

'Your span of life, complexion, strength, health, lustre and energy are the result of your digestive fire.'—Swami Sivananda

Our gurus have emphasized the paramountcy of fire in the phenomenal world. In the Hindu tradition, fire is revered as being sacred, a bridge between the physical and the subtle worlds. In all the significant rituals of the human lifecycle, we perform fire rituals. *Homas* are performed during rituals of birth, marriage and death. Fire is perceived as *sakshi*, a divine, incontrovertible witness to all our rites of passage. Likewise, Ayurveda too holds that fire bears witness to all the processes of the mind and body, acting upon it in a fundamental, life-giving way.

If one were to gaze contemplatively into a fire, the obvious question that ought to arise is why fire is hot. Yet, people seldom ponder the 'whys' in nature and its phenomena. If we looked closely, we would see that fire is a magical form of energy that drives momentum into objects. It moves, transforms and regenerates what it touches. Agni or fire is the third of the five great elements (panchbhuta) of the visible cosmos. According to Ayurveda, fire unfolds from ether and air, and that the agni element is the very energy turbine of our constitution. Hence, we call it the fire of life.

Agni runs an amazing system of governance across our body: it produces digestive enzymes, controls digestion, absorption and assimilation (which is further responsible for the production of ojas and tejas, vital energies that we will discuss in depth later), runs all metabolic activities, supplies nutrition to our tissues and maintains body temperature, complexion, vitality and vigour, apart from sharpening our visual perception to enhance mental clarity.

Agni reconstructs the cytoplasmic content of food into consciousness and keeps our minds nourished at a cellular level. It acts upon the nuclear membranes of cells, nourishes our genes and DNA and acts as the guardian of our genetic code. Thus are all the cells of our body conserved and nourished, and the cellular metabolic activities smoothly governed. Agni ensures that our tissues mature and sustain themselves in tune with our daily living.

In addition to the above, agni nourishes our intelligence, keeps our cells in perfect communication, arms us with courage and confidence and gives us a sense of discrimination and a clear logical perspective. When our cellular intelligence works perfectly, we are assured of a normal body temperature, a healthy complexion and above all, pure contentment. Therefore, agni, the digestive fire, is the nucleus of health.

Digestive enzymes turn the food we ingest into the energy we need. The action of agni turns whatever we eat into biological elements. However, the action of agni is not only biological—it also transforms food into textures of consciousness. Any food we eat also has the five elements. To optimally nourish our body tissues, food particles have to be not only absorbed but also enjoyed, because the sensual experience is an important aspect of nutrition.

It is agni that drives both these processes—the sensory as well as the assimilatory. When you bring food near your mouth, the mind at once registers which biochemical catalysts are needed for this particular food and the appropriate secretions take place in the mouth. This will trigger the particular aspect of *jatharagni* (digestive fire) needed for that food. Just as agni rules digestion, it also rules the process of excretion, the final exit point of the digestive process. It governs urinal, faecal and sweat-related excretions. It keeps what the body needs and throws out what is unnecessary. This is why agni is also called the gatekeeper. When our agni is in perfect balance, we will naturally have a sensible approach to food, with an absence of greed or unhealthy cravings.

Agni rules not just food and digestion but also all our sensory perceptions. Every sensory input that we receive as sound or touch or taste or smell has to be 'digested'. Therefore, agni is the force that governs our essential understanding of the outer world. Conversely, if our agni is imbalanced, it leads to not just bad digestion of food, causing bloating, constipation and diarrhoea etc., but also leads to utter chaos in our sensory receptors, resulting in depression and emotional disturbance.

Traditionally, Ayurveda recognizes thirteen types of agni depending on its function and site of action. Among these, jatharagni is held as being of primary importance. It is the gateway to all the other aspects of agni at work in our bodies. Jatharagni is present in the stomach and duodenum. It is responsible for the maintenance of rasa, dosha, dhatu and mala—the various processes and constituents of the body. It stimulates and augments the five *bhootagnis* (the agnis present in the five elements in our bodies) and the seven *dhatvagnis* (agnis present in the dhatus or tissues in our body).

It is vital that we nourish, balance, regulate and nurture our digestive fire. Anything that goes in through our mouth or even our skin is monitored, broken down and processed by the force of agni. Even the Ayurvedic medicines taken orally and applied on the skin etc. are processed through the force of agni.

Ayurveda is very clear that an impaired agni is the root cause of all diseases. Now, what is it that impairs the agni? A bad diet, a harsh lifestyle, reckless habitual patterns etc. lead to a sustained state of stress and emotional turbulence, which in turn results in a disruption of agni power.

An unhealthy lifestyle aggravates bodily doshas and imbalances the agni in the body. For instance, modern lifestyles, where people eat late, sleep late and wake up late, are habits that are highly detrimental to our natural agni. The fact is that the dynamic properties of our inner agni are directly linked to the solar cycles. The 'sun clock' is directly related to our 'agni clock'. A fundamental precept of Ayurveda emphasizes this law. It says that we are a microcosm of the universe. That which is in the universe is also within us.

The ancient text *Yajur Veda* states:

> '*Yatha pinde tatha brahmande*' meaning 'As the individual, so is the universe'.
> Charaka, the preceptor of Ayurveda, writes, '*Purushoyam loka sannidah*', meaning 'Man is a miniature universe'.

At noon, when the sun is closest to the earth, our agni power is highest. That is the time that is best for having your heaviest meal of the day. When the sun goes down, our agni power drops and therefore, eating a very light meal after sunset is recommended.

A poor state of agni leads to the opposite of well-being. A weak agni could cause impaired visual perception manifesting as corneal opacity, cataract, glaucoma or iritis. It could bring about fatigue, indigestion, bloating, constipation, hyperacidity and a general feeling of congestion of body and mind. It makes a person susceptible to fears and anxieties. It could discolour the skin, making it pale. The modern mind fails to make the connection between the earth's cycles and our state of mental and physical health.

For instance, a damaged agni could result in inner conflicts and a loss of courage, which in turn could cause a person to flee situations and relationships. Even a young person could feel lethargic or lazy and find it hard to cope with deadlines. Even worse, a diminishing agni may cause a person to feel like withdrawing from life. As the vital fires burn low, it drains a person's capacity to digest life experiences and thus the aging process is accelerated.

Ayurveda urges us to reclaim our agni power. To do this, it is necessary to first identify the elements that are imbalanced in our system. A certified or accredited Ayurvedic physician can help us identify our agni problems.

4

The Power of Flavour

Rasa, virya and vipak

Ayurveda has a unique approach to nutrition. It addresses the body's reaction to food rather than just the nutrients in the food itself. What that means is that an individual's unique experience of a particular food will determine its nutritional value to that person.

This is done through the classification of the three processes of rasa, *virya* and *vipak*, which can be understood as taste, power and post-digestive effect. These three help predict the therapeutic qualities of a particular food for a particular individual. When food or any liquid is placed on the tongue, rasa is the first experience. After swallowing, and as it enters the stomach, *virya* is the hot or cold sensation that follows. How the body feels within the first couple of hours of partaking a particular food determines the virya or power

Table 2: The rasas

Rasa (taste)	Predominating elements	Characteristics	Found in	Function	Excess can cause
Sweet (Madhura)	Earth plus water	Cooling, oily, heavy	Carbohydrates, fats, protein, rice, wheat, sugar, honey, liquorice, dairy products and sweet fruits like dates, mangoes etc.	Balances vata and pitta. Strengthens body tissues, enhances ojas, has soothing effect on nerves, benefits the skin, promotes longevity	Aggravation in kapha. Diabetes, obesity, lymphatic congestion, lethargy, build-up of ama (toxins)
Sour (Amla)	Earth plus fire	Hot, light, oily	Foods that have citric and ascorbic acetic acid. Fruits like amla, lemons and vegetables like tomatoes; yoghurt, vinegar, alcohol, pickled and fermented foods	Balances vata. Helps in appetite and digestion, blood circulation, eliminations of waste from the body. Good for heart and brain.	Imbalance in pitta and kapha. Acidity, heart burn, ulcers, rise in temperature, itching, blood toxicity, sensitivity of teeth and allergies.

Rasa (taste)	Predominating elements	Characteristics	Found in	Function	Excess can cause
Salt (*Lavana*)	Water plus fire	Hot, moist, heavy	All salts like sea salt, black salt, common salt and mineral rock salt (*saindhava* or *sendha namak*)	Balances vata. Maintains electrolyte balance, stimulates salivation, enhances appetite and growth, strengthens muscles, provides radiance to skin, helps in the functioning of the digestive system, laxative	Aggravation in pitta and kapha. Hypertension, oedema, peptic ulcers, vomiting, excessive thirst, skin wrinkling and skin problems

Rasa (taste)	Predominating elements	Characteristics	Found in	Function	Excess can cause
Pungent (*teekshna*)	Air plus fire	Hot, dry, light, anti-spasmodic, anti-parasitic	All essential oils. Foods like asafoetida, mustard, garlic, onions, ginger, hot peppers	Beneficial for kapha, stimulates metabolism, purifies blood, improves blood circulation and sensory perception, helps in losing weight, promotes sweating, clears sinus passages, aids in deworming	Imbalance in vata and pitta. Irritability, nausea, diarrhoea, muscle pain, weakness, fatigue
Bitter (*kadwa, katu*)	Air plus ether	Cool, light, dry, anti-parasitic, antiviral, antibiotic	Foods with alkaloids. Bitter gourd, neem, radish, basil, fenugreek, broccoli, turmeric, dark green leafy vegetables, coffee	Harmonizes pitta and kapha. Purifies blood, helps in liver aliments, obesity, nausea, fever and in cleansing the system	Aggravation in vata. Negative effect on bone marrow and semen, reduction in sexual energy, dehydration, emaciation, dryness, gas, constipation, insomnia

Rasa (taste)	Predominating elements	Characteristics	Found in	Function	Excess can cause
Astringent (Kashaya)	Air plus earth	Dry, cool, heavy	Foods rich in tannin. Tea, arjuna, pomegranates, green apples, green grapes, green beans, cauliflower, okra, cabbage, coriander, turmeric, alfa alfa sprouts, lotus seeds	Good for pitta and kapha. Helps in inflammatory conditions, decongestant, cleanses mucus membranes and clears ama.. Maintains healthy blood sugar levels, promotes healing and blood clotting, eliminates excess fat	Aggravation in vata. Insomnia, spasms, gas, constipation, dryness and thirst

of that food on the body. Vipak is the post-digestive effect of the substance consumed and the long-term value or effect of the food on the body.

There are six tastes or rasas and each is composed of two of the five elements. There is a deep relationship between each taste and its two predominant elements.

Making healthy choices

To make the right choice of food, we should consider our particular 'dosha constitution' and seek expert help in deciding the best food for us. It is recommended that all six rasas be incorporated in your meals as far as is possible. Ideally, three meals a day are suggested. Breakfast and lunch should be hearty meals, given the relationship of the 'agni power' with the sun. Needless to say, it is best to eat organically grown fruits and vegetables as they naturally clean our digestive system, besides providing safe nourishment.

Lunch should be the most sumptuous meal of the day, because at noon agni tatva, the fire quotient within us, is at its peak when the sun is at its hottest. Our agni tatva increases and decreases in direct proportion to the rising and the setting of the sun. If we are inclined to indulging in heavy or fried food and desserts, lunch is the best time to consume these. Our body will handle the absorption with more fire power.

Dinner should be had no later than 7.30 or 8 p.m. Harmonize your diet in a manner that the dinner intake sees you through to breakfast and the breakfast food sees you through to lunch and the lunch menu sustains you well till dinnertime. We should avoid snacking, but considering our current erratic lifestyles and untimely hunger, small quantities of healthy snacks between meals is recommended. Suggested snacks are a small bowl of poha or upma or spiced puffed rice, foxnuts, a couple of pieces of dhokla or a fistful of nuts or a fruit.

Fruits and dry fruits are hydrating, cleansing and important sources of dietary fibre. Being rich in vitamins and minerals, they form a protective shield against many diseases. Fruits are most beneficial to us when eaten as per the appropriate season. Ripe, sweet and fresh fruits require little digestion to convert into nutritional fluid. Hence, the ideal time to take fruits is approximately two hours after breakfast and an hour before lunch or two hours after lunch and an hour before sunset. If we eat fruits along with other cooked foods, they go through 'over-digestion' and get fermented, which results in the formation of ama (flatulence). It is to be noted that melon is suggested as a stand-alone fruit, meaning it should not be consumed along with any other fruit or food. Ayurveda recommends that rather than eating melons along with other foods, it is better not to eat them at all. When it comes to dry fruits, it is advised to soak them overnight in water or milk and then consume them.

For an adult, it is important to have at least two servings of fruits or dry fruits daily. One serving of fruit is one medium-sized fruit or two small fruits or one cup of diced fruits. The ideal one-time serving of dry fruit is 50 grams. It is good if a couple of more servings can be accommodated.

Dietary guidelines as per your dosha

Vata type

People with a vata constitution need oil, ghee and butter in their diets. Therefore, they may indulge in fried foods and rich foods.

Vegetables recommended are those that belong to the gourd family, especially parwal (pointed gourd), lauki (sweet gourd), torai (ridge gourd), pumpkin, lotus stem and radishes.

Fruits, dry fruits and spices recommended for vata constitutions are apple, pomegranate, custard apple, ripe mangoes, bael or quince, dates, raisins, foxnuts, hing (asafoetida), black pepper, cumin, fennel, Indian gooseberry (amla), mint and basil.

Flaxseeds may be added to their food liberally.

Vata people should consume brown and red rice and millets.

Foods to be eaten sparingly by vata types are peas, leafy vegetables, lentils, potatoes, peanuts and extra sour fruit.

Vata types should avoid fasting, excessive use of purgatives, or an excess of sex, running or any form of exercise.

Pitta type

Pitta types need a preponderance of sweetness in their diets. It is recommended that they include ghee, jaggery and natural sugars such as honey, dates, barley and crystallized sugar in their diet.

Vegetables recommended are radish, water chestnut, bottle gourd, petha (ash gourd) and pumpkin.

Fruits and spices that suit pitta types are ripe bananas, sugarcane, fresh coconut, watermelon, custard apple, grapes, raisins, fennel, coriander, chironji (an almond-like seed also called the Cuddapah almond), psyllium husk, natural rock salt and cardamom.

Beverages such as cold milk, sugarcane juice, buttermilk, aloe vera pulp, coconut water, amla juice and sherbets made from khus, rose and sandalwood extracts are recommended for the pitta body type, including water that has been stored in an earthen vessel. Fresh curd is also beneficial to the pitta-predominant body type.

Foods to be eaten sparingly are sour curd, sour buttermilk, brinjals, drumstick, bitter gourd, jackfruit, ragi, bajra, chillis, asafoetida, peanuts and oily foods.

Pitta people are sensitive to sunlight. They should never fast or go hungry or be deprived of sleep. They are particularly advised against smoking tobacco.

Kapha type

Foods that have astringent, spicy and bitter qualities suit the kapha constitution. Flavours that are sour, salty and sweet should be consumed sparingly.

Astringent foods include vegetables such as Brussels sprouts, broccoli, cabbage, carrots, cauliflower, green beans, turnips, alfa alfa sprouts, bell peppers, onions, lettuce, peas and fruits such as apples, cranberries, pomegranate and avocado.

Spices and herbs, such as ginger, cardamom, mint, basil, tea, coffee, Indian gooseberry, figs, saffron, black pepper, garlic, red and green chillies, cloves, fenugreek, turmeric, cumin, ajwain (seeds of ajowan caraway and kalonji (nigella) are recommended.

Foods for the kapha-predominant person to eat sparingly are pumpkin, milk and milk products, coconut and coconut water, tamarind, ber (Indian jujube), unripe guava, oils of almond and sesame and chironji.

Important tips for healthy eating

Some recommendations apply to all body types—for instance, freshly harvested new grains should not be consumed. Grains such as rice, lentils, wheat and millets should be appropriately stored and aged before they are consumed as these are heating in nature and can lead to vata and pitta imbalances.

Mangoes should always be soaked for at least two hours before consumption in order to reduce their heat element. Refrigerating them does not have the same effect.

With the exception of the apple, no fruit should be eaten on an empty stomach, i.e., first thing in the morning. Papayas should never be eaten on an empty stomach. Fruit should never be eaten during or soon after a meal—with the exception of banana, papaya and pomegranate. Other fruits are best eaten sometime between breakfast and lunch. No fruit should be eaten after sunset.

It's better not to snack through the day. It is best to simply take three good meals.

Avoid cold drinks and carbonated drinks. Instead, make it a habit to sip warm water through the day. It will fuel your agni.

Do not stand while eating. Avoid watching videos or using the phone or even reading while eating, so that you ingest the food consciously and mindfully. Chew your food well, letting your taste buds experience the various rasas of the food. Enjoy whatever you are eating. Your mood sets in motion the digestion and absorption of your food. Have a solid lunch. At night, drink soups or eat salads or have a very light dinner. Let eating food be like a 'prayer in motion', where one gives thanks at the outset of the meal and gratitude at the end of it.

Avoid all packaged foods. As far as possible, avoid eating reheated or stale food. However, stale and reconstituted chapattis are good for you. Incompatible food combinations are a *big* no (see box below).

Fast once in a while, perhaps on Sundays or on holidays when you are not working. In case you are unable to fast, you could switch to soups or broths or herbal tea. You could also opt for water fasting, single-meal fasting or juice fasting as you like. Or you could simply have only khichdi (a gruel of overboiled rice and pulses) for the day. Such periodic and regular dietary cleansing will certainly aid the agni in your body.

Most importantly, loosen your mind and live light-hearted and happy. You will be surprised at the extent to which your state of mind determines your digestion.

A traditional cure for chest congestion

Two teaspoons of pure cow ghee mixed into a quarter cup of warm milk is a wonderful remedy for congestion. Taken once or twice a day on an empty stomach and continued over a few days, this simple home remedy is guaranteed to clear the most persistent chest congestion. Do not eat or drink anything for an hour after administering.

Incompatible food combinations

Certain foods should never be taken together as they could result in putrefaction, fermentation or indigestion. The following food combinations are not recommended:

- Milk in combination with any citrus juice.
- Fruit should never be eaten during or soon after a meal, with the exception of banana, papaya and pomegranate.
- However, papaya and pomegranate should not be taken together.
- Milk and non-vegetarian food items. It is advisable to wait a minimum of seven to eight hours after eating fish, chicken or red meats before consuming milk.
- Milk and curd.
- Milk and radishes.
- Melon should always be eaten alone—neither with any food nor with any other fruit.

- Tea/coffee/hot drinks should not be had with yoghurt.
- Honey should never be heated or added to any food or drink that is piping hot.

Balmarogyamayushch pranashchagno pratishthita
Annapanendh naishchagnirjwalati vyeti chanyatha (342)—
Charaka Samhita

Strength, health, longevity and vital breath are dependent upon the power of digestion, including metabolism. When supplied with fuel in the form of food and drink, this power of digestion is sustained; it dwindles when deprived of it.

5

The Three Pillars of Ayurveda

'Yabhih kriyabhir jayante sharire dhatava samah,
Sa chikitsa vikaranam karma tad bhishajam smritam'
—*Charaka Samhita*

('This is a holistic science using whatever means is effective
to restore balance to the body and mind')

Ayurveda describes food, sleep and sex as being the three
pillars of life, or the *tri-stambha*. Each is dependent on the
other and they are all intertwined in their relationship with
ojas, the subtle essence that rules our immunity, vigour and
vitality, which in turn keep us emotionally and spiritually
healthy. If one of these three pillars is disturbed, it will have a
damaging effect on the other two pillars, and this in turn will
dilute and deplete ojas.

Food: the fine art of eating

Hippocrates, the ancient Greek physician traditionally considered to be the father of medicine, wrote: 'Leave your drugs in the chemist's pot if you can heal the patient with food.'

An Ayurvedic proverb expressed the same many centuries before him: 'When the diet is wrong, medicine is of no use. When the diet is correct, there is no need for medicine.' What is good health if not a perfect state of equilibrium within one's self? We must be aware of the invisible bond between the microcosm and the macrocosm before we understand the Ayurvedic idea of food as medicine. The intimate connection of not just food, but also the source of the food with the seasons, the environment and local geography, is not overlooked by Ayurveda's astonishing wisdom. Of course, modern medicinal science has its own nutritional concepts. But Ayurveda has had a very deep epistemological understanding of these things from very early times. Contemporary science is now advancing towards the holistic perception that Ayurveda has held for centuries.

For instance, physics today has begun to accept the idea that everything in the cosmos is interconnected. Yet, even so, it limits this interconnectedness to the physical. Ayurveda goes much further. According to Ayurveda, it's not just about what we eat and when we eat. How food behaves in our bodies is determined by subtle, non-physical factors. For instance, how did we earn the money to buy the food? Did we earn it ethically or is it money earned dishonestly? In short, a good, nutritious diet doesn't start from the kitchen; it starts from our source of household income. In what mood were we when we bought grains, pulses, vegetables or fruit? Is the cooking space clean and peaceful? What was our state of mind when we cooked the food? Our bodies are as spiritual as they are physical and all these subtle influences act upon how we receive and digest our food.

Ancient wisdom urges us to recognize the quality of our energies. Our income is the creative output of our energy. If earned by fair means, it becomes imbued with *sattvic* energy; if earned through unfair practices, it carries with it an energy quotient that will not be beneficial to us, whether we are consciously aware of it or not. If money has been earned through dishonest means, it carries *rajasic* and *tamasic* vibrations into the food purchased, which is then transferred into our bodies. This is the holistic approach of Ayurveda to food.

It is also important to calm our mind when we are shopping for food. We must pay a fair price and do so happily. Too much bargaining is best avoided, for such energy then attaches itself to the food, sending anxious and irritated vibrations into our bodies when we consume it.

Likewise, food must be cooked in a place that is clean, peaceful and hygienic. The cooking too should be done in a spirit of love and nurturing. In olden times, in India, it was common for the mother or whoever was cooking to chant mantras or sing devotional songs while cooking. This would infuse the food with powerful waves of sattvic energy that had the power to heal and nurture all who partook of it.

August Turak, a well-known entrepreneur, studied the business success of a group of Trappist monks of the Mepkin Abbey in South Carolina. He noted that hundreds of grocers, caterers and bakers were willing to go the extra mile to buy fruitcakes, cheese, mushrooms and even eggs from the Mepkin monastery. He discovered that the secrets of their success were the important ingredients that these pious old men added to their products: 1) selflessness 2) ethics and 3) faith in love. Turak went on to write a bestselling book, *Business Secrets of the Trappist Monks: One CEO's Quest for Meaning and Authenticity*, about how our complex body-mind system is nourished through food blended with the energy of miracles!

When it comes to nutrition, it is important to allow the satva guna to dominate. Fresh fruits, vegetables, grains, pulses and milk products all have the satva quality. There are also foods such as potatoes, tomatoes, sour fruits and some spices that are rajasic in nature. Most overripe fruits, mushrooms, eggs, stale food, non-vegetarian food etc. are tamasic and should be carefully balanced in one's diet. Ayurveda sometimes prescribes tamasic food in small quantities when it acts as a medicine. For example, if you lack protein, you may consume egg whites, chicken or fish. Additionally, many fermented foods such as curd, dosas, idli etc., though categorized as tamasic, are rich in friendly bacteria, promoting gut health and increasing our agni energy. These constitute an important part of a balanced diet. Once we have diagnosed our body type, we can design a meal plan in which the satva guna dominates.

Today, we are seeing a trend towards genetically engineered or modified foods. Ayurveda has always emphasized the importance of living in synchronicity with the magnificent and flawless design of nature. The *bija* or gene of every plant has evolved in perfect consonance with the grand design of the cosmos. Each bija is a unique, intuitive and flawless expression of the cosmic intelligence. Therefore, extreme caution must be exercised and sustained trials conducted before genetically modified foods are introduced into our diets.

Organic plants contain ojas, tejas and prana—their innate forces of energy. The use of chemical insecticides and hormones depletes these energies in the plant and they fail to nourish us sufficiently. Inevitably, large quantities of these toxic substances find their way into our diets, often with tragic consequences. Recent decades have seen an exponential increase in tumours and cancers as our bodies are bombarded by toxic substances. Ayurveda suggests the use of natural fertilizers and insecticides, such as cow dung and neem derivatives. Humans are only custodians of nature and certainly not its owners. Well-being lies in living in harmony with nature.

Water: the source of life

'Water is Life's matter and matrix, mother and medium. There's no life without water.' —Albert Szent-Gyorgyi, the discoverer of vitamin C

Water, the fourth element, is the source of life. Wherever there is water, there is the possibility of life. Over 60 per cent of our bodies is water. Here's a quick break-up: according to H.H. Mitchell of the University of Illinois (*Journal of Biological Chemistry*, v. 158, issue 3, p. 625–63)., our brains and heart are made of 73 per cent water. Our lungs are about 83 per cent water and 64 per cent of our skin is water. Muscles and kidneys are 79 per cent water. Even our bones are 31 per cent water. Water is present in our body as plasma, cytoplasm, serum, cerebrospinal fluid, sweat, urine etc. Water hydrates tissues and cells, assists digestion, balances our pitta dosha, enhances kapha whenever needed and lubricates vata. Water also regulates our body temperature. It heals our body of fatigue, nourishes our skin, increases our stamina and pacifies *sadhaka pitta* to strengthen our heart.

A well-hydrated body functions well and keeps the mind calm. It keeps common headaches and constipation at bay. Water by itself is a natural method for detoxification. Often, our hunger may not be for food, but thirst for more water. Drinking a glass of water causes hunger pangs to subside. Water controls the flow of neurological impulses, moistens the surfaces of joints, smoothens the respiratory system and supplies fluids to support the pleura and pericardium membranes that support the lungs and the heart, respectively.

Ayurveda says that depending on our age and gender, we must drink a liberal amount of water daily. An adult male should take in a minimum of about 3 litres, while an adult female may drink at least 2 litres every day. If we pay attention to the needs of our bodies, we should drink water as soon as we experience thirst and stop when we feel contented. Summer afternoons are the hottest pitta time and extra water is needed to stabilize our body temperature. Of course, some of the required water will come from the food we eat. Our needs will vary according to our constitution. Vata and pitta types might need more water than kapha-dominated constitutions.

Ayurveda recommends that water be boiled with added spices to cleanse our *srotas* or micro channels. Pitta pacifiers like lemon, rose or mint leaves can be added where needed. Boiled and cooled water is better received by our bodies. An experienced vaid can recommend a water recipe based on a person's constitution. Appropriate spice water recipes help balance each of our doshas and cleanse our systems. If we drink an insufficient amount of water, it will manifest as dry skin, constipation, weight loss and weakness in the reproductive tissues.

Followers of New Age movements, influenced by a metaphysical understanding of nature, have propounded that water is a medium of divine consciousness. This is supported by studies showing that water molecules organize themselves into geometric designs. These patterns/formations are now known to hold energetic imprints from activities, influences and even thoughts to which the water has been exposed. In effect, it is proven that water has 'memory'.

Dr Masaru Emoto in his bestselling book *The Hidden Messages in Water* cites frozen water crystal photography to prove that water responds to our thoughts and feelings. He demonstrated how, when water is blessed or verbally loved or touched or cared for by humans, a charming symmetry takes shape in its molecular structure. Conversely, if the water is cursed or exposed to anger or any negative emotion, the molecules take on dissonant dysmorphic forms. The Russian physicist Konstantin Korotkov in his paper on 'Study of structured water and its biological effects' has demonstrated how even small changes of projected mental intention can change the quality of water.[3]

Indian yogi Sadhguru Jaggi Vasudev also reiterates this: 'Much experimentation has been done and they have found that water has memory—it remembers everything that it touches. Our grandmothers used to say we should drink water or eat food received from people who love and care for us. Because water remembers the divine. This is an important part of what "Teerth" (pilgrimage) is. People want to drink water from a sacred site so that it reminds them of the divinity within. The same H_2O can become poison or the elixir of life, depending on the memories it carries.'[4] Therefore, water must always be approached with care, love and responsibility.

Drinking water sensibly

The practice of drinking water as soon as we wake up is called *ushapan*. It cleanses our intestines, flushes out toxins from the previous day, balances the doshas and stimulates digestion.

We should drink water either at room temperature or boiled and cooled. Warm water helps unblock our arteries and balances cholesterol levels. On the other hand, cold/chilled water dulls the agni and hampers the digestion process.

Water should be drunk in a smooth manner and never gulped down. If possible, sit and drink (as opposed to standing) for best absorption.

It is advised to have water half an hour before meals. If needed, water may be sipped during meals but not taken immediately after meals (unless it is hot water). We may again drink water 45 minutes after a meal if required.

Store water in copper (*tamba*) or silver (*chaandi*) vessels. Drinking such water helps to balance our body's doshas. Copper is an essential mineral that is known to have antimicrobial, anti-inflammatory and antioxidant properties. When water is stored in a copper vessel for eight hours or more, it releases some of its ions into the water. Copper pacifies kapha and kindles agni. Similarly, silver too has the power to remove free radicals from the body, cooling the intestines and aiding digestion. Silver pacifies the pitta dosha. The properties of gold are proved to pacify vata and pitta dosha.

Water may also be stored in a clay pot. Not only does this cool the water naturally, but the clay increases the alkalinity of the water, thereby maintaining the pH balance and keeping acidity at bay. Water should be stored in a clay pot only in summer, when its properties are beneficial for all doshas. In winter, water from a clay pot will aggravate the kapha dosha.

Water may also be spiced with tiny pieces of ginger, slices of cucumber, mint leaves and drops of lemon juice, etc.

Sleep

The divine gift of sleep

> 'Happiness, misery, nourishment, emaciation, strength, weakness, virility, sterility, knowledge, ignorance, life and death—all these occur depending on proper or improper sleep.' —*Charaka Samhita*

Of the human activities fundamental to health, sleep is the one that is most commonly compromised in modern lifestyles. Internet and social media addictions are common in both the young and the old. Long working hours and even socializing late into the night eat into time that ought to be set aside for sleep. Insufficient sleep has disastrous consequences, especially on the young. Children who were good at studies suddenly begin to slide or those who were sweet-tempered start becoming aggressive and angry. Many start to eat more and gain weight abnormally. There is an increasing number of children being diagnosed with diabetes or high blood pressure, diseases hitherto restricted to the old. Sleep deprivation quickly leads to depression, diabetes, high BP, obesity and cardiovascular disease. Unless these sleep debts are compensated for, we will be forced to pay a high price. Our long-term strength, potency and intelligence depends on the quality of the night sleep we get. Inadequate sleep leads to disturbance of our prana. If sleep is not smooth and deep, the gastro-intestinal tract gets clogged with ama or undigested food, blocking the flow of prana. Similarly, untimely and excessive sleep can also steal happiness away from our life.

A recent study conducted by the Department of Neurology, National Institute of Mental Health and Neurosciences (NIMHANS), Bengaluru, India on sleep disorders found that about 210 of 1050 healthy men and women in south India had significant sleep-related problems. Some suffered from sleep apnoea with choking and some experienced excessive sleepiness during the day. It was found that sleep deprivation led to depression, morning headaches, sleep paralysis, cataplexy with physical collapse, insomnia, anxiety and hallucinations. Many were found to be struggling with sleep initiation and maintenance as well. It is obvious that sleep disorders will eventually weaken the immune system and lead to severe health issues.

Sleep is one of the three most important pillars of the art of perfect living according to Ayurveda. Sleep is the best state of mind-body relaxation. According to the Dalai Lama, 'Sleep is the best meditation.' Each day, our perceptions are converted into functional intelligence. In our waking hours, the mind is being constantly bombarded by sensory inputs and an endless stream of information. The mind digests this flow of data to create coherent thoughts, emotions and experiences. To achieve an optimal state of mind power, we need to give our mind proper rest in the form of sound sleep.

Our brain actively passes through five stages to give us a complete sleep cycle. The first stage is a shallow and light sleep followed by the second stage, which represents deeper sleep. The third and fourth stages of the sleep cycle are progressively deeper stages of sleep. These last two stages of sleep are called Slow Wave Sleep (SWS). The fifth and last

stage of the sleep cycle is Rapid Eye Movement (REM) sleep
and is associated with dreaming and sleep-walking. REM is
believed to be the stage where memory consolidation takes
place and the mind-body system is able to recuperate and
rebuild itself.

One sleep cycle lasts about 90 minutes. So a good night's
sleep would be one that gives five to six cycles of sleep. In
a sattvic person whose doshas are more balanced, sleep will
be deep and sound. The sleep of a rajasic person will often
be light and interrupted by disturbing dreams. A tamasic
person, on the other hand, tends to sleep for longer hours,
even during the daytime. *Alpanidra* or sleep deprivation and
atinidra or over-sleeping are both not good for our health.
The recommended sleep time for an adult is seven to nine
hours, though some schools of thought prescribe six to eight
hours. Young people under eighteen are advised to sleep for
eight to ten hours every night.

Thought suggestion about sleep starts in the mind and is
felt in the late evening. So the activities we engage in late in
the evening will tend to affect our night sleep pattern. If our
evening activity is calming, even if it be a noisy, vibrant party,
we are likely to experience a sound sleep that night. Ayurveda
recommends that we take a short time to sit undisturbed in a
pleasant mood before we go to bed. This helps the mind exit
from the day's stresses and tension. The quality of our sleep
is closely connected with our state of mind. Sleep being one
of life's most important activities, our preparation for sleep
should be accorded equal importance. Our sleep should be
in perfect rhythm with the sun's cycles. Short power naps

during the day are okay, but sleeping during the sunset hours should be avoided.

Ayurveda's guide to perfect sleep

The sun is man's best guide to eating and sleeping. Simply put, we should rise with the sun and prepare to sleep after the sun goes down. We are a solar-powered planet and by aligning ourselves to the sun's rising and setting schedules, our personal rhythm will synchronize with that of nature. The circadian rhythm is our natural body clock which, if left undisturbed, will regulate our sleeping and waking cycles, repeating itself every twenty-four hours.

Ayurveda attaches great importance to the way we sleep. While eight hours of sleep is recommended at night, it is also fine to take a short siesta after lunch, especially on hot days. Generally, it is said that sleeping on one's left side aids digestion while sleeping on the right side promotes relaxation. But for each dosha type, a particular sleeping position can be recommended. Sleeping on one's stomach is never recommended as it obstructs deep breathing. Intake of food should be avoided for at least two hours before we go to bed as sleeping on a full stomach diverts the body's energy towards the process of digestion. When we allow the body time to digest a meal before sleeping, the body's energies work towards relaxing and recharging the system.

The well-known Indian mystic Sadhguru advises a lukewarm bath or shower before going to bed. This is to not only cleanse the dirt from the body but also to wash away unwanted thoughts from our mind. According to him, a bath or shower has a natural tendency to release tensions and make us alert. Seventy per cent of our bodies are water, and so when we run water over it, a certain purification (*shuddhikaran*) happens, which goes well beyond the mere cleaning of the skin. Sadhguru also suggests lighting a small lamp with a cotton wick soaked in any organic oil and chanting a mantra before we sleep. If, before sleeping, we spend 5–10 minutes to ponder the constructive actions of the day and then set them aside, we will find ourselves waking up with renewed potential energy to solve the challenges of the new day.

Impact of doshas on sleep

As individual doshas determine everything about a person, sleep quality is also affected by the doshas in different ways. Vata types will naturally find it difficult to get into a calm mode. Their minds are always excitable and active. So they are advised to take short naps to calm their senses. When vata is predominant in our dosha type, then the individual needs to work towards 'calming habits' in order to get a good sleep. Vata type people need to take extra care to not feel cold when they sleep. Further, if the sleep is insufficient for a vata person, it leads to an even higher vata level, which in turn weakens body tissues. Pitta dosha people, on the other hand, exhibit an amazing amount of energy around midnight. This is because their agni levels are proactive and high even after the sun goes down. They have a good digestion even if they eat late. Pitta types tend to get almost uninterrupted sleep, even though their sleeping time is of medium duration. To calm and relax their mind, pitta types can elect to read or meditate before sleeping. Kapha type people also sleep well, provided they follow healthy habits. If they sleep too much, it increases the kapha dosha, which causes weight gain and lethargy. Kapha types need to check their tendency to indulge in excess sleep.

Food affects sleep

What we eat will also affect our sleep. A modest intake of sweets is good as the sweet rasa brings tenderness and softness into our bodily energy, which will help promote sleep. However, we must be careful to not overdo this. A small quantity of lukewarm milk at bedtime is also recommended. At dinner, one should avoid excess meat, yoghurt and cheese. This is because these substances increase the *medha* dhatu (fat) and provoke our kapha unnecessarily, resulting in a slowing of metabolism and an increase in lethargy and oversleeping.

Sleeping on our side

It is fascinating to note that if we consciously follow the right sleeping habits, our bodies will naturally change their positions through the night, in ways that promote the correct chemical balance.

Our right side holds the solar or masculine force field, while the left holds the lunar or feminine force vibrations. Here, when we use the terms 'masculine' and 'feminine', we are not referring to gender but to two complementary aspects of a whole. People who habitually choose to sleep on their left side are seen to suppress their lunar energy and aggravate their solar energy, creating an excess of pitta. People who always sleep on their right side will find that their solar energy gets suppressed. Ayurveda recommends that pitta people sleep on their right as much as possible. By suppressing their solar side, their pulsating agni energy can be slightly subdued as they need more calmness. Sleeping on the right side calms the pitta nature. However, if followed for a long duration, this will result in an increase of kapha, leading to congestion in the sinus. Sleeping on an oversoft bed or a water-bed could also lead to an escalation of kapha. And again, sleeping on too hard a surface will result in an increase of vata. A middle path, as always, is best. Vata and kapha types should opt to sleep on their left side. This helps the bigger part of the belly go down while the upper part presses onto the liver, stimulating an acidic secretion, which aids digestion.

Sleep and the directions

The direction in which we place our head while sleeping is critical to our well-being. Ayurveda expressly prohibits sleeping with our heads pointing to the north. Leading Ayurveda expert Vasant Lad goes to the extent of saying that 'only dead people sleep pointing north'.[5] A custom prevalent among Hindus is of laying a dead body with the head pointing northward. The reasoning for this is that the human body, as a microcosm of the earth, can also be said to have its own magnetic poles. When you place the positive ends of two magnets together, they will repel each other and vice versa. In the human system, the head can be said to be its positive pole. For those who live in the northern hemisphere, therefore, it is recommended that they never sleep with their head facing the geographic north as it will exercise a strong magnetic pull on the human system. This pull affects blood circulation, resulting in stress and illness, including strokes and haemorrhage at worst or disturbed sleep at best.

Sleeping with the head pointed east results in better focus and sharper memory. It promotes a tranquil, meditative and refreshing sleep and consequently a healthy mind and body. Sleeping with our head pointed to the west and south are considered auspicious. In accordance with the magnetic pole theory, for those in the northern hemisphere, when the feet are towards the north and head towards the magnetic south, there is a harmonious mutual attraction that draws energy into the body, bringing success, wealth and fame into our lives. The ancient Indian architectural science of Vastu Shastra also supports these Ayurvedic concepts and recommends placing sleeping spaces in the south, east, west and south-west of the house. It is practical to experiment with these sleep directions for a few weeks and discover for ourselves which sleep direction works best for our body-mind constitution.

Sex

The sacred stairway to the self

'A man practicing *dharma, artha* and *kama* enjoys happiness both in this world and in the world to come.' —*Kama Sutra*

Sex is sacred. While it is the highest form of bodily pleasure a human can enjoy, sex is also considered as being a doorway to self-realization. Only sex or *maithuna* offers us the mighty experience of the sacred amalgamation of male and female energy. This fusion of energies far transcends the physical. Our ancient texts say that, during the act of maithuna, the couple experience the metaphysical union of Shiva and Shakti tasting the ultimate reality and experiencing bliss. In effect, sex is an act of spiritual transformation.

Unfortunately, sex often gets a bad press because of the moral inconsistencies that invariably attach themselves to sex. However, if kama is practised within the framework of dharma, this primal drive for pleasure reveals itself as being one of nature's most profound existential truths.

Ayurveda considers sex as being one of the three vital pillars (tri-stambhas) of health and an expression of the creative life force in action. Like food and sleep, sex too needs to be approached consciously. It asks us to regularly review how efficiently these three segments of our life are functioning. Are they improving our health, vitality and creativity? Or are they draining our vigour and leaving us fatigued?

Of the three pillars, sex is the highest form of the lowest energy that resides in our root chakra. It is important to guide this energy and direct it appropriately to deepen our connection with our partners and also with our higher self. This is owing to the divine bio-psychological power of sexual fulfilment. Along our spinal cord runs an ascending and descending subtle channel that carries pure pranic energy along the seven chakras or energy centres. The muladhara or the root chakra, located at the base of the spine, is considered to be the seat of sexual energy.

According to Vatsyayana, author of the *Kama Sutra*, the iconic treatise on sexual behaviour, 'The ability to create maximum pleasure in a partner and exploring these pleasures is the key to maintaining love and balance of power between two partners.'[6] In the matrix of our life, sex becomes the 'agent procreator' of the species. Nothing other than the sexual drive can ensure a continuum of life forms on our planet. The German psychoanalyst Sigmund Freud had identified that an instinctual drive for pleasure, called 'libido', drives all human actions. He believed that humans possess an instinctual libido from birth and that it expands in five stages. But this was widely misunderstood as a mere sex drive. By the term libido, Freud actually meant much more. In this context, libido is to be viewed as life force or prana. Of course, physically it is also manifested as the sexual drive. But that is not the whole story. Libido can take on a whole array of forms to express a galaxy of experiences. A few thousand years before Freud, Ayurveda taught us that the sexual impulse is present all over in a human body. Every cell, it said, is a 'sex cell'.

'Without food and clothes, the body becomes thin and weak. Without eroticism, the mind becomes restless and unsatisfied.'[7] Let us understand how the three interconnected pillars of food, sleep and sex build up our life.

i)   Nourishing food and ample sleep together ensure that we get enough daily functional energy.

ii) This leads to a sustained amount of healthy libido, which acts as the essential creative life-force in us.

iii) Sex and creativity are expressions of a healthy libido, which in turn are the foundations of a happy, healthy and fulfilling life.

Thus, all three together, food, sleep and sex, work in harmony to maintain health and well-being.

Understanding the dynamics of sexual union

Sex is the most dynamic form of prana and is the catalyst of creation and creativity. Nonetheless, this sacred energy is often defiled by cultural taboos and conditioned mindsets. Parents need to guide their adolescent children on understanding, accepting, celebrating and channelizing their sexual urges. Studies show that a vast majority of human conflicts are directly or indirectly related to the suppression of sexual needs. If sexual energy is traumatized or blocked, it can lead to emotional imbalance, psychological disturbances and physical health problems.

When two individuals love each other and, within that loving relationship, engage in sex that is aware and conscious, they gain the ability to transform their ojas into bliss. Here, a mere ejaculation or orgasm is not the goal. It is a prolonged and joyful pleasuring of each other that fills the partners with physical, mental and spiritual contentment, emphasizing the love flowing beneath the act. As this conjugal bonding grows stronger, it leads to a higher degree of harmony in all aspects of their relationship. Just as a conscious mode of living is recommended by Ayurveda, a conscious and aware engagement of mutual pleasuring (in sex) is also recommended. It increases the love of two souls for each other.

Maintaining our vitality

Now for an understanding of the Ayurvedic perspective of the biology of sex: of our seven layers of skin, the deepest layer is the *shukradhara kala*, the membrane that is responsible for sexual desire. Shukra dhatu is present throughout the body. For instance, if the lover takes hold of the hand of his or her beloved and caresses it lovingly, it naturally and easily results in sexual arousal. Even if he or she were to look deeply into the eyes of the beloved or exchange a meaningful glance, desire flares up. This is the work of the shukradhara kala.

The male and female organs have similar functions, but look deeper and we will see the dialectics of nature: if the male sperm is cold, alkaline and active, the female ovum is hot and passive. This is diametrically opposite or a mirror view of the cosmic perspective where Purusha is passive and Prakruti is active. Through such intelligently designed dialectics, mutual attraction is assured and the chemistry of creation continues eternally.

The sex organs are directly connected to the root chakra, which is also the location of the dormant *kundalini shakti*. If this power is suffocating in the root chakra, a person may get crazily addicted to sex. If we elevate this shakti towards the call of love, sexual union can foster a constructive energy that is beneficial to the individual. This energy, if properly channelled, has the potential to act as a springboard to enlightenment. Even if it does not, it allows even an ordinary person to have a foretaste of the divine. The act of sex, when performed in a spirit of pure love, blurs the boundaries of the self, creating a sense of boundlessness and spiritual bliss. However, pure love and surrender are absolutely necessary for this to happen. On the other hand, when sexual energy remains trapped in the muladhara, people tend to masturbate and this consequently leads to the diminishing of his or her ojas.

Having sex with the right partner, in the right frame of mind and at the right time, has the power to charge the root chakra. Emotions play a very important role in intercourse. Anxiety, fear and anger are detrimental to our sexual appetite. These need to be cleansed from our mind before engaging in sex. During sex, a certain amount of ojas or vital energy is used up. Since ojas is the foundation of immunity, therefore it is advisable to take measures that help regenerate ojas. Obviously, overindulgence in sex can lead to depletion in ojas and this will further damage the immune system An imbalance or any disturbance in shukra dhatu rasa can create sexual fatigue or weakness. Therefore, all dhatus and rasas should be nourished with the right food and supplements. Foods with excess pungent and bitter vipak can also deplete sexual energy, reducing sexual secretions, like semen, and causing problems in their discharge.

Ayurveda suggests that the role of sex, apart from procreation, is also to foster creative energy in our lives.

Hence, it is helpful to cleanse our root chakra through meditation, mudras and mantras.

Sex and body types

The physical constitution plays a big role in sexual habits. Vata types are romantic but erratic in nature. They enjoy foreplay, caressing and being caressed. Soothing music and a light oil massage escalate their desire. Ayurveda advises them to take rejuvenating drinks regularly. Pitta types have a natural zest and zeal for sex. They like to dominate during the sexual act and also tend to vent suppressed feelings through it. Ayurveda advises them to channel their passion through the emotions of love, care and sensitivity towards their partner. They should avoid excessive sex. Kapha types have ideal qualities for lovemaking when adequately motivated. They are endowed with affection, sensuality, sensitivity and endurance. They enjoy giving pleasure and are gentle with their partner.

Sex and the seasons

The acceptable frequency of sexual activity varies from person to person and from season to season. With regard to frequency, Ayurveda emphasizes the principle of *ritucharya*, i.e., synchronizing our living to the rhythms of nature. Here, the seasons play a vital role in our sex lives. Winter *(shishir ritu)* is when the body is at its most vital and hence, that is the best time for frequent sex. In spring *(vasant ritu)* and autumn (*sharat/hemant ritu*), our stamina is moderate, so sexual frequency should also be moderate. In the rainy season (*varsha ritu*) and summer (*greeshm ritu*), the bodily strength is at its lowest, so lower frequency of intercourse is prescribed.

The ideal time for sex is two hours after dinner and two hours before midnight. Food needs to be properly digested before the act so that energy is at its optimal level. A light dinner followed by sweet desserts is ideal. It is to be noted that having sex soon after meals is harmful to the body system. In fact, sex is best avoided both after heavy meals as well as when we are hungry.

The best day of the month to have sex is on the full moon night after 10 p.m. Additionally, Ayurveda proscribes having sex when a woman is menstruating. It also prohibits sex during pregnancy or soon after delivery.

The right ambience for sex

'Kama is the enjoyment of appropriate objects by the five senses of hearing, feeling, seeing, tasting and smelling, assisted by the mind together with the soul.'—Vatsyayana, *Kama Sutra*

Where and how to have sex is also important. The act of sex must be seen as the opening of the gates of the mind to receive another body-mind complex into itself with love. To enhance our receptivity, we must consciously cleanse ourselves of negative thoughts and enter into a pleasant and positive mood. This will directly affect the quality of lovemaking. Ecstasy is only possible when both partners are in a conducive frame of mind.

Creating a pleasurable ambience in the room through soft lighting is suggested as it is pleasing to see the responses of one's partner during the act. Likewise, a sensual, enticing aroma in the room can be created by placing fragrant flowers by the bed. Soothing music will enhance the romantic atmosphere. A shared bath with aromatic oils and salts before sex will have the effect of increasing mutual desire. Extended foreplay is strongly prescribed in order to assure the partner of their importance. Self-confidence is critical to sexual bliss. There is no need to follow any prevalent porn culture, which can lead to unrealistic expectations and feelings of anxiety and inadequacy. Instead, the mood should be caring, tender and relaxed. The purpose of all these prescriptions is to enable the shedding of all inhibitions, both personal and cultural, so that the partners can surrender themselves wholly to each other, to their own sensuality and partake of what is the most delightful and precious human experience.

Sexual positions and partners

Vatsyayana's *Kama Sutra* describes sixty-four basic positions for making love. Among these, Ayurveda gives greatest importance to the missionary position, the most common sexual position in which the man lies on top of the woman to engage in vaginal intercourse, both in terms of pleasure and for the purpose of conception.

With regard to one's partner, Ayurveda recommends sex only within a committed relationship in a spirit of trust and loyalty. As it is said, the best aphrodisiac is the right partner.

Ancient perspectives on homosexuality

Ancient India accepted homosexuality as an acquired human tendency prevailing in societies. Texts like the *Kama Sutra* affirm and recognize same-sex relations and many Hindu temples have carvings that acknowledge alternate sexual orientations.

As for Ayurveda, it simply accepted the reality of having a third stream of sexual orientation among humans. The *Sushruta Samhita* sketches certain male and female profiles who are aroused only through feelings for the same sex. Male minds identified as *kumbhika* experience pleasure only through anal penetration while *asekya* type of men find pleasure by offering oral sex to other males.[8] Charaka writes of women who develop sexual feelings for other women owing to a genetic effect of vata of the mother's ovaries on the embryo.[9]

6

Prana and Ojas: The Awesome Twosome of Immunity

A humane and radical aspect of Ayurveda is its honesty of approach in not attempting to suppress the symptoms of disease. Rather, it is a healing system that is ever watchful of symptoms and focuses on addressing their root cause right down to the level of the mind. Illness is identified as a sign of the depletion of dynamism in the body-mind complex. Therefore, attacking the symptoms is superficial. Ayurveda aims at identifying the cause behind the symptoms and activating the patient's own immune system to overcome the malady. Disease is akin to a burglar alarm going off. No sensible person will attack the alarm—instead, they will try to spot the burglar. Similarly, if we have a disease, Ayurveda studies the vital area of our system where the anomaly has developed and identifies the underlying cause. Accordingly, it activates our immune system. It recognizes immunity as supreme in restoring and maintaining health.

Immunity depends on factors as varied as proper digestion, powerful agni, smooth functioning of the liver and a well-balanced endocrine system that ensures a perfect balance of hormones. However, beyond all these visible, traceable factors lies the ultimate secret of our immunity—ojas. Though the word 'ojas' literally means 'vigour', the subtlety of ojas makes it a mysterious, intangible essence in our bodies. Ojas is the very foundation of immunity. The state of our ojas determines our state of health. Therefore, in order to understand the secret of immunity, we need to understand ojas.

Ojas, our mysterious guardian
Vartyanti Prinita sarvadehin
Yadyate sarvabhootanam jeevitam navtishthate
—*Charaka Samhita*

'Ojas keeps all living beings nourished and refreshed. There can be no life without ojas.'

Ojas is the pure, superfine sap of life energy. As ghee is the purest essence of milk, ojas is the subtlest and most concentrated, superfine extract of energy resulting from perfect digestion. It is the purest subtle essence present in all our bodily tissues. When it is present in its full capacity as per our constitution, we stay well and healthy, and when it is harmed or diluted, we can fall ill in the same proportion. Ojas could be termed as the 'source fluid' that runs and governs all our physical capabilities.

Ojas is formed from the biosynthesis of bodily tissues. Once the food we eat has been completely digested, *ahar rasa*, the nutritional extract, is formed. This nutrient, once absorbed into the digestive tract, is synthesized by the digestive fire to form the first of the seven tissues, rasa dhatu or plasma, which in turn carries it to the other dhatus. The last distillate of the biosynthesis of all the dhatus is ojas. Ojas, as the superfine biological end-product of digestion at the cellular level, is the most powerful guardian of our immunity. Hence, we must ensure a high ojas quotient for a healthy life.

Ojas energises the immune system. If vaccination is an acquired immunity factor, ojas is our natural immunity factor. The strength of our ojas determines whether internal or external threats are capable of causing a disease. When ojas is strong, it will fight and block harmful viruses and bacteria.

Apart from our food, our ojas quotient also depends on the quality of our thoughts and lifestyle. Happy relationships, a pleasant environment and a regular routine act as a potent tonic for our ojas. Ojas is also influenced by the quantum of agni in our system. If agni is in optimal condition, it can be said with certainty that our immune system is strong.

How doshas affect immunity

Immunity can also be diluted by an imbalance of vata, pitta and kapha. When we suffer from 'chronic fatigue syndrome', it could be due to pitta stagnating in the concerned nerve endings, which in turn affects the immunity of our majja dhatu (bone marrow), nerve tissues and connective tissues. In such instances, it is advisable to seek pitta treatment to correct our immunity levels. A high level of pitta has a tendency to burn ojas and could make one susceptible to autoimmune diseases.

Ojas, tejas, prana

The body is sustained by two fundamental facets—breath and food. Breath and food together create the tissues of the body and the thoughts of the mind. Both are transmuted into cosmic essences, which Ayurveda differentiates as ojas, tejas and prana.

Just like the three doshas, ojas, tejas and prana are also made up of the five elements, except that they exist in the most subtle form in an individual. The subtle essence of kapha dosha is ojas and relates to the water element in particular. The subtle essence of pitta dosha is tejas and relates to the fire element in particular. Vata dosha's subtle essence is prana, which relates to the ether element. Every cell has its own intelligence that comes from tejas, while ojas is responsible for its vigour. Prana is responsible for the flow of intercellular intelligence.

Expressions of tejas

Tejas expresses itself in physical form (*rupa*) as the radiance of the skin, the brightness of the eyes and the strength of the bones and muscles etc. We experience the sensation of touch as an expression of tejas in cellular intelligence. The multiplication of cells that form new tissues is also determined by tejas. It is also tejas that is responsible for our sense of perception, for instance, our ability to see in a three-dimensional manner. Tejas is responsible for the ability of cells to differentiate. For instance, if there is an abnormal growth in our tissue or the formation of an ulcer, tejas recognizes it and separates it as an anomaly. Further, tejas constructs our body mass by uniting the molecules of similar quality through attraction. Even the suitable quantum of fat that needs to be accumulated is an expression of tejas. Tejas, together with prana, has the amazing ability to liquify and expel toxins from our body. Tejas and prana further control cellular *gati* or movement. Natural urges such as sneezing, urinating, defecating, sweating etc. are all a result of the gati power of tejas and prana.

Prana, the force of life

Literally, 'prana' means 'breath'. It is that and much more. It has many levels of meaning, from the physical breath to the flow of energy within the human body, to the energy of consciousness itself, each level more subtle than the last.

Within the human system, it is understood as the subtle form of vayu dosha. The following are the five types of vayus within us: (i) prana vayu (ii) apana vayu, (iii) samana vayu (iv) udana vayu and (v) vyana vayu. These five are involved in the assimilation, distribution and management of all the different types of energies needed for body functioning. The pranas are responsible for respiration, oxygenation and circulation. It is the pranic force that kindles the subtle agni and the natural, spontaneous intelligence of the body cells. The pranas govern our sensory and motor functions and all physiological functions. Prana also governs the higher activities and functions of our mind—our memory, thoughts and emotions. Prana operates in an intertwined manner with ojas and tejas.

The human body has a bilateral symmetry—like our right and left arm, our right and left ear. Basically, most of our organs have two balanced parts—for instance, the testicles, the ovaries, the kidneys, the lungs etc. As we know, the right side of our body is governed by our left brain and vice versa. Ayurveda defines the right side as solar, which is male. The left is considered lunar, which is female. Prana balances the dynamics of these dual systems. The polarity of positive and negative energies in us is bridged by prana, which is both masculine and feminine. Prana, through respiration, bonds the male and female energies within us. Respiration is not just a mechanical activity. It has its own mind, feelings, direction and enthusiasm. This is because our prana is synchronized with the cosmic prana. When we inhale, outwardly it appears as if we are inhaling air, but in reality, our prana is also drawing life energy from the universal cosmic prana. When we exhale, our individual prana goes out into the cosmic field. Prana is a magnificent gift that sustains our life itself.

7

Transcending Sexual Urges for Spiritual Ascension

While Ayurveda shows us how to celebrate sexual union in the finest possible way, it also points towards what lies beyond. Those in the throes of sensual pleasures would have difficulties with ideas of celibacy and *brahmacharya*. But the reality is that sex is only the outward expression of the divine capacity of our libido. Ayurveda also teaches that by transcending our sexual urges, we can gain astonishing capabilities and a reward of total bliss.

The experience of sex has a powerful impact on our mind and bodily system. While Ayurveda writes extensively about the benefits of healthy sexual activity, it emphasizes equally the importance of moderating our cravings and sensibly guiding them towards higher goals. According to Swami Sivananda, the great proponent of Vedanta and yoga, if men and women restrict sexual indulgence to mere procreation, then that itself is observance of brahmacharya. Total abstinence is enjoined on those who seek the higher values of life. Till such time as a strong inner urge towards abstinence arises, it would be futile and self-destructive to fight the cravings of libido, because that would amount to fighting the very essence of life. It begins with exercising discrimination and putting checks and balances in our sexual behaviour. This kind of self-control will offer us a superior state of balance in our mind, speech and behaviour.

Once a person reaches a stage of sexual satiation and fulfilment, their libidinal energy can be utilized as a path to self-realization. Realized masters say that mental and spiritual ascension awaits us once we have fulfilled the necessary imperatives of kama, karma and dharma. A totally contented yogi, who has gone beyond sexual urges, can utilize their sexual energy as a path to *samadhi* or the final union with divine bliss.

Brahmacharya

Brahmacharya is a widely misunderstood concept. It literally means 'conduct consistent with the path of Brahman', the ultimate reality. It is characterized by sexual abstinence but is fundamentally different from the western understanding of celibacy, which is limited to non-indulgence in sex. Brahmacharya instead focuses on restraint of the mind. It means plugging ourselves into the greatest force field available to mankind. Patanjali's *Yoga Sutra* says: 'On being

established in celibacy, vigour is gained.'[10] The preservation
of semen boosts our self-confidence and increases our inner
capabilities. None other than the Advaita Vedanta Mahaguru
Sri Sankaracharya spoke of the astonishing power of semen
retention:

> To the celibate who conserves the semen,
> what is there unattainable in this world?
> By the power of composure of semen,
> one will become just like one's self.[11]

Semen in its subtlest form is called ojas and pervades every
cell of our body. It has been proven that semen retention
increases the testosterone level. In addition to increasing our
IQ, it also helps control our moods and levels of motivation.
By transcending, as opposed to suppressing, the pleasure urge
and retaining our sexual energy, specifically the semen, we
are able to harness mighty powers of mind, body and speech.
Our powers of retention, willpower (manobal) and immunity
increase dramatically. It opens our mind to intuitive wisdom
and faculties to which we normally do not have access. Our
spiritual capacities expand and our perceptions deepen
radically. In effect, we become wiser, more profound beings.
Yogis and ascetics in India traditionally observe brahmacharya
for many years or all their lives. It has been observed that the
longer the period of brahmacharya, the more ojas and atma
virya or spiritual energy increases.

It is important to understand that the transmuting of
the semen's energy into ojas and tejas does not pertain only

to men. Women who practice brahmacharya transmute the reproductive energy that produces the ova and the menstrual cycle. These energies are transformed into ojas and tejas exactly as in men. When a woman practices brahmacharya, she has the potential to control her reproductive energies.

Semen is the finest pranic extract of all bodily functions. It is said that just as water, when channelized correctly, has the power to become electricity, so semen, when directed properly, charges and energizes the body dramatically. According to Ayurveda, brahmacharya is potentially the elixir of eternal youth.

The celebrated Guru Paramahamsa Yogananda remained a virgin all through his life. He died in the US in 1952 in the middle of delivering a lecture, with a beatific smile on his face. Days after his death, his body remained fresh, causing an uproar around the world. Mr. Harry T. Rowe, Los Angeles Mortuary Director of Forest Lawn Memorial-Park Association, in a notarized three-page letter wrote, 'The absence of any visual signs of decay in the dead body of Paramahansa Yogananda offers the most extraordinary case in our experience. No physical disintegration was visible in his body even twenty days after death. No indication of mold was visible on his skin and no visible drying up took place in the bodily tissues. This state of perfect preservation of a body is, so far as we know from mortuary annals, an unparalleled one. No odour of decay emanated from his body at any time.' Ayurveda attributes this 'miracle' to his state of perfect brahmacharya.

Similarly, Swami Vivekananda, another celebrated Indian monk, was able to read and retain large books within a matter of a few hours. He had a photographic memory and had the ability to quote precisely from them without a single error. To his astonished audience, Vivekananda explained: 'By observing brahmacharya, all learning can be mastered in a short time.'[12]

Sadhguru Jaggi Vasudev describes brahmacharya as being a kind of *sadhana* or spiritual discipline. It can be understood as an internal maintenance technique whereby the practitioner makes sure that no energy is wasted, and one becomes energy conscious.[13]

Please note, brahmacharya should be undertaken only under the tutelage of an experienced teacher. Effective brahmacharya involves prescribed diets, controlled lifestyles and spiritual practices.

8

Tackling Obesity through Ayurveda

Let us begin with clearing a misconception: Fat is not evil. It is widely believed that fat refers to unwanted weight in the body. In modern times, it is considered a curse. This is far from the truth. Fat or medha is one of the seven dhatus or building blocks of the body. Fat is the body's fuel. It plies and plays between joints, acting as the perfect lubricant and moving them smoothly. Fat allows muscles to move freely without friction. Fat stores energy and releases it when required, keeping our bodies healthy and firm. A moderate amount of fat is necessary for every individual. Insufficient fat results in dry and rough skin and damaged joints.

Vasant Lad says: 'There is fat on round organs, such as kidney, liver, spleen, heart and diaphragm. Behind the eyeball there is fat, because the eyes are the body's most active organs. They are constantly moving and need lubrication and nature has provided fat to give them freedom of movement . . . Fat is necessary to nourish the glandular system—the thyroid, parathyroid, adrenals, ovaries and pituitary. Medha dhatu is also related to perception. Superfine molecules of medha dhatu help the brain retain healthy and blissful memories.'[14]

According to Ayurveda, fat is predominantly a blend of earth and water. These elements add bulk and strength to our body. When there is an imbalance in our doshas, our agni is affected and this results in an accumulation of ama (undigested food). When our jatharagni is not in balance, the sequential formation of the seven dhatus (body tissues) is disrupted and their respective agnis are affected. This results in a build-up of ama and toxicity in the body. In time, this results in obesity. Only when the jatharagni is strong can it enable the dhatvagnis to function properly.

Ayurveda terms obesity as *atisthaulya* or *medha roga*, which means an excessive accumulation of medha (fat). Medha along with mamsa (muscle) together become lard, turning the body flabby. Let us examine the lifestyle reasons behind obesity. Obviously, overeating along with poor nutrition top the list. Excess intake of kapha increasing foods, such as salt, sugar, dairy products and sweets, or foods that take longer to digest, such as red meats, are the prime reasons for weight gain. Alcohol, drugs and steroids, which are rich in water and earth molecules, also cause obesity. A sedentary lifestyle, comfort-eating, prolonged stress and anxiety and unresolved emotional residues in the mind contribute to obesity. Incompatible food combinations are another reason. Then there are factors, such as metabolic disorders, weak digestion (*mandagni*), hormonal imbalances, genetic disorders and even hereditary factors.

There are instances when obesity is not caused by food alone. It could also be caused by depression. Sometimes, people are more depressed during the winter due to the lack of sunlight and tend to overeat. Ayurveda emphasizes the importance of sunlight to our wellbeing; the lack of it can certainly cause anxiety or depression, a condition classified as Seasonal Affective Disorder (SAD).

Heredity also plays an important role in perpetuating obesity. Ayurveda says that our DNA carries the biochemical memory of our parents' illnesses and physiological/psychological conditions. If parents or grandparents or even great-grandparents were obese, one's cells are bound to carry the memory of this. Even food habits and cravings of ancestors within two generations are found to be handed over to children.

The state of our liver is the foremost factor to consider when addressing obesity. The secretions of each organ contribute to the process of metabolism. When one's liver suffers a fatty build-up, it is indicative that the cells of the liver are struggling to metabolize fat molecules. The fat molecules then accumulate in the liver as unmetabolized fat and may result in an obese body. Alcohol is another cause of abnormal medha dhatu. Though alcohol is easily metabolized by the liver, excessive consumption of alcohol can create fat deposits, as the liver converts alcohol into sugar. Since alcohol is fermented sugar, it kindles jatharagni, which could cause alcoholics to eat more than necessary. This could put them on the road to obesity.

Obesity has universally been identified as being a deep-rooted psychological problem. The discrepancy between what the body requires and psychological cravings for food needs to be understood. It is not necessarily the body but the mind that creates emotional cravings, which are interpreted as a desire for chocolates, sweets, fried food or alcohol, etc. If we become aware of our thought processes, these misinterpretations can be kept in check. Our physical constitution or dosha may be set at birth, but the power to alter our mental attitudes remains with us.

In a simple way, Ayurveda suggests it is advisable to divide the capacity of one's stomach into three parts: one part for food, one part for water and one part for air. If one eats to full capacity, one is not leaving the desired space for air and water. This tendency to eat to one's capacity could also be a form of emotional/comfort eating, which means that physiologically, one doesn't need that much food for the body.

Ayurvedic guide to reversing obesity

'For every ailment known to man, God has given us a plant to heal it.'—*Vannoy Gentles Fite*

Ayurveda gives us many wonderful ways to address obesity. It recommends certain herbs to improve the power of agni at the tissue level itself. Thrikatu, guggulu, daruharidra, calamus (vacha), barberry, kutki, chitrak, shilajit, arjun, catechu, karanja and ativisha/atees and other herbs are recommended to be taken as per one's constitution under expert guidance.

If one is suffering from troubles caused by ama, specific herbs that strengthen the power of agni to dissolve ama are prescribed. These are chitrak, fresh ginger/dry ginger (sonth), black pepper, guduch and turmeric.

Ayurveda states that foods that have the following rasas have a tendency to reduce fat:

Tikta rasa (bitter) helps scrape away and remove the accumulation of fat. *Katu rasa* (pungent) kindles the digestive fire and helps to cure obesity, abdominal swelling and excess fluid retention. *Kashaya rasa* (astringent) alleviates kapha. *Amla rasa* (sour) kindles the digestive fire as it liquefies kapha.

Anti-obesity herbs

According to Ayurveda, the following herbs aid in tackling obesity.

Garcinia Cambogia: Commonly known as Malabar tamarind or *vriksha amla*, this fruit lowers the appetite, aiding in fat metabolism. It inhibits the synthesis of fats and lipids and decreases the formation of LDL cholesterol along with triglycerides. The hydroxycitric acid in the fruit rind of garcinia blocks the production and storage of fat and cholesterol in the blood whenever the calorie intake exceeds the levels of healthy eating.

Guggulu: This is a kind of resin that has fat-burning properties and controls cholesterol and triglycerides.

Mustaka: Commonly known as nutgrass or nagarmotha, it reduces fat deposits, stimulates digestion and works as an astringent.

Triphala: This is a popular ayurvedic formulation composed of amla (Indian gooseberry), haritaki and bahera. It helps in discharging waste products from the body through urine and faeces. It cleanses the colon naturally and detoxifies the body. It further aids in reducing constipation and works to enhance bile secretion, which aids in metabolism.

Ginger (Zingiber officinale): Ginger is considered to be the most sattvic and the best of spices. It aids in stimulating the jatharagni, thereby improving the digestive process.

Sunthi (dried ginger) has a hotter characteristic then fresh ginger. It is a stimulant and an expectorant used for decreasing kapha and increasing agni.

Pippali (Piper longum): This is a powerful stimulant for the digestive system as it removes congestion and ama.

Trikatu: (Kali mirch + sonth + pippali) possesses the unique quality of rejuvenating agni and burning away ama.

Bilva (bael) (aegle marmelos): This is considered one of the most sacred plants in India. It is an important astringent and stimulant that improves malabsorption and weak digestion. It improves both the digestive fire and the function of the small intestine.

Chitrak (Plumbago zeylonica): This herb is most effective in strengthening the digestive fires in the liver, small intestine and spleen. In certain cases, it works better than trikatu.

Turmeric (haridra, Curcuma longa): This spice promotes metabolism, strengthens digestion, heals and improves intestinal flora and particularly aids in the digestion of proteins.

Guduchi (Tinospora cardifolia): This parasitic creeper rejuvenates pitta. Its hot nature acts against the ama in one's body.

Garlic (Allium sativum): Cleanses ama and kapha from the blood and lymphatic system.

Haritaki (Terminalia chebula): The name of this herb derives from the word 'harna' or carrying away of all diseases. It regulates kapha, cleanses the colon and corrects constipation and/or diarrhoea.

All of these must be taken in correct doses under expert supervision. Overdosing may lead to toxicity.

More methods to banish obesity

Panchkarma therapy is highly recommended for weight loss. This therapy has five fundamental processes which, among other curative effects, also guides the movement of ama, bringing it back to the digestive tract and then expelling it from the body system. Panchkarma therapy should only be done under the guidance of an expert vaidya.

Massage is referred to as *abhyanga*. When massaged with certain herbal powders/pastes/oils, fat deposits (medha) are 'broken' and expelled from the body. Massage is excellent for improving blood circulation and toning the muscles, provided it is done correctly using oils suited to one's constitution.

Apple cider vinegar helps in maintaining metabolism. Drinking two teaspoons mixed in a glass of water are advised. However, not all remedies work for all. It's best to do this under expert supervision.

One teaspoon honey and the juice of one or half a lemon mixed in lukewarm water consumed daily helps in reducing fat accumulation.

Upavasa (fasting) at least once a week improves one's metabolism as the body, when deprived of food, readily utilizes fat already stored in the body.

Consuming cold beverages and foods is to be avoided as these tend to aggravate kapha and douse agni.

Obesity has universally been identified as being a deep-rooted psychological problem. The discrepancy between what the body requires and psychological cravings for food needs to be understood.

9

Spices: The Wonder Foods

In Ayurveda, spices are called the 'wonder food'. In India, every geographical region specializes in spices that grow best in that particular soil and climate. Wherever one lives, one will find the spices best suited to their gut. Each regional microculture knows which spices are most suited for them. Spices in general play an important role in stimulating agni. Some are best had sauteed in ghee, others can be dry roasted or eaten raw or simply added to foods.

(i)   Kali mirch or black pepper improves agni. It enhances the secretion of digestive juices and aids in destroying toxins. It is especially good for kapha and vata-natured people. Pitta-dominant people should use it sparingly.

Freshly ground pepper can be sprinkled on vegetable salads or fruits. If you sprinkle it on any fruit/vegetable/

food, it has the effect of enhancing the nutritional qualities of that food item.

(ii)   Adrak or ginger is called the 'universal medicine'. Its pungent taste has excellent digestive absorption qualities.

It is also ideal for our respiratory system as it helps to neutralize toxins in our body. It is very useful for an aggravated kapha and vata-natured people. Pitta-dominant people should use it sparingly. Health expert Anthony William, in his book *Liver Rescue*, explains that ginger is key to liver health. It balances the liver and feeds it with dozens of phytochemical compounds that expel ammonia and rotten, putrefying foods and debris. It dislodges fat cells from the liver and purges them through the bile and digestive tract.

(iii) Hing or asafoetida is one of the key spices for aiding digestion. It curtails flatulence, helps in metabolism and is an excellent source of antioxidants. It is recommended for vata and kapha-natured people. Pitta-natured people should use it sparingly. The combination of hing and cumin in curries and lentils is very good for digestion.

(iv)   Zeera or cumin is a powerful diuretic and a digestive. Cumin helps digestion and clears the flow of urine. Cumin increases the release of bile, which helps the functioning of the liver and pancreas. It is also naturally rich in iron.

(v)   Sabut dhania or coriander seeds act as a soothing balm to a disturbed digestion. It whets the appetite and benefits the digestive enzymes. It is also an excellent diuretic, balances the doshas and is therefore good for all body types. In India, it is a common custom to take a *mukhwas* or mouth freshener after meals. Mukhwas usually includes whole spices, such as coriander, to aid in digestion.

(vi) Ajwain or ajowan caraway is excellent for digestion. It also has aphrodisiacal properties, besides being an antibacterial, anti-fungal agent. It is good for vata and kapha-natured people. Pitta-natured ones should use it sparingly.

(vii) Haldi or turmeric enhances metabolism and aids in detoxing the liver. It is a unique antioxidant and has healing, anti-inflammatory and anti-allergic properties. Particularly recommended in the winter, it is suited to all body types. Turmeric is widely used in various curries and dishes.

(viii) Saunf or fennel stimulates the digestive fire without aggravating pitta. It is excellent for digestion and suited to all body types. Fennel can be dry roasted and stored.

(ix) Methi seeds or fenugreek aid in treating digestive disorders and have healing properties. It is beneficial in treating joint pains and also helps in maintaining the blood sugar levels.

(x) Dalchini or cinnamon pacifies disorders of the stomach and aids digestion. It also aids in stabilizing blood sugar levels and is good for all body types.

(xi) Elaichi or cardamom aids in digestion, assimilation and circulation. It tends to help clear mucus in the stomach and is recommended for all body types.

(xii) Sarson or mustard seeds imparts strength and combats dryness within the system.

(xiii) Laung or cloves stimulate digestion while calming the pitta. It is anti-fungal, antibacterial and rich in antioxidants. It promotes liver and bone health and is said to have aphrodisiacal properties.

(xiv) Chakra phool or star anise has anti-spasmodic, antiviral and anti-ageing properties. It is good for digestion and is helpful in managing diabetes.

Yogvahi is a unique concept in Ayurveda, which recognizes certain foods as being yogvahi, meaning that they act as bioenhancers. A bioenhancer is an agent which, while having its own pharmacological properties, also enhances the efficacy and absorption of other therapeutic substances with which it is co-administered. The word yogvahi literally translates as 'synergism', i.e. the action of increasing the efficacy of a substance by another unrelated substance. For instance, using yogvahi agents, such as honey or ghee, together with certain herbs will carry the qualities of those herbs to all seven dhatus. Yogvahi is therefore the hallmark of polyherbal formulations in Ayurveda.

In Ayurveda, the following are considered to be yogvahi:

i) Honey

ii) Black pepper

iii) Dry ginger

iv) Cow ghee

v) Guggulu, a particular kind of gum resin

vi) Asphaltum or shilajit

These can be incorporated into our daily diets to enhance the properties of our food. However, keep in mind that honey should never be added to hot substances.

Simple home remedies with common spices

i) Just about 30 minutes before lunch, if an inch-long piece of ginger is chewed slowly, it will give rise to extra saliva, which in turn increases the jatharagni. A pinch of salt can also be added to the ginger—the combined rasa of ginger and salt will spark the jatharagni even better.

ii) A decoction made by boiling a piece of ginger, crushed black pepper pods and a few Indian basil leaves (tulsi) is an excellent remedy for coughs, colds and seasonal flu.

iii) Make a mixture of whole almonds soaked in just enough honey to bind and add a liberal dash of crushed black pepper. This can be stored and eaten every day. Since both pepper and honey are yogvahi foods, they enhance the nutritional value of the almonds exponentially.

iv) A simple cure to alleviate stomach discomfort and gas is to apply a paste of hing powder mixed with water around the navel.

v) Soak a teaspoon of cumin seeds in a glass of water at night and drink it in the morning to benefit from its diuretic effect. If you boil the water, the cumin becomes more potent. The use of cumin is widespread in Indian food culture. Being rich in iron, it is traditionally given to lactating mothers in various forms to increase the flow of milk.

vi) In India, fennel is customarily eaten after meals as mukhwas. When it is chewed bit by bit with the saliva, its benefits increase manifold. A teaspoon of fennel soaked in water overnight and taken in the morning is a healthy habit.

Make your own Ayurvedic mukhwas by making a mixture of 2 tbsp. roasted fennel, 2 tbsp. roasted white sesame seeds, 2 tbsp. roasted coriander seeds, 1 tbsp. roasted flax seeds, ½ tbsp dried coconut powder and 2 tsp. cardamom seeds. You can add some rock candy to taste.

vii) A quarter teaspoon of ajwain and a pinch of salt in a glass of lukewarm water is excellent for digestion. It relieves indigestion, flatulence, nausea and colic pain. Salt can also be substituted with rock candy.

Ajwain is also used for massage. A few tablespoons of ajwain tied in a piece of soft muslin is dipped in warm oil and used for massage to aid in improving muscle tone, digestion and skin health. This kind of massage is traditionally done for postpartum recovery.

viii) Turmeric is ubiquitous as a remedy in traditional Indian households. Turmeric boiled in warm milk and a little water is used as a healing, antiseptic tonic.

A mixture of turmeric and warm cow ghee is an excellent remedy for cuts, bruises and skin disorders.

In the olden days, a warm poultice of turmeric and cow ghee was applied inside a woman's vagina after childbirth. This aided in quick healing and prevention of infections.

viiii) A heaped teaspoon of soaked or germinated methi (fenugreek) seeds are advised to be taken with water or tea. Methi is good for maintaining healthy joints as well as being beneficial for managing diabetes. Methi laddoos made with ghee are very popular in many Indian states.

ix) If you are a coffee drinker, it has been found to be beneficial to brew a little cinnamon powder with your coffee. This offsets the edginess induced by the caffeine and balances the mood.

x) Clove oil is an excellent remedy for toothaches.

10

Herbs: The Wonder Drugs

Modern science is only just beginning to align itself with traditional medicine, as biochemistry and empirical evidence validates what the compendium of Charaka stated over 2000 years ago. Knowledge of the medicinal properties of herbs and how they interact with the human body was a science perfected by the preceptors of Ayurveda. In fact, it is a science far more sophisticated, more complex and more precise than modern medicine. Modern medicine treats the illness whereas Ayurveda treats the individual. What this means is that Ayurveda does not believe that one size fits all. Instead, individuals are classified according to their personal doshas, which means the unique way they interact with their environment, their unique psychological traits and their unique genetic predispositions. Based on this classification, they are then prescribed a unique treatment tailored precisely to their needs.

In the same way, Ayurveda states that herbs and minerals impart their healing properties through their unique guna (qualities), rasa (taste), virya (energy), *prabhava* (effect) and vipak (post-digestive effect). Their properties will also vary depending on the terrain from which the herb/mineral was sourced, the season and even the time of the day. The properties will further vary depending on how it is prepared—whether boiled, dried, crushed etc. The properties will further vary depending on what is prescribed in conjunction with it. All these layers of complexity were understood and compiled by the ancient fathers of Ayurveda.

Some commonly used herbs and minerals prescribed in Ayurveda are:

1. Ashwagandha (*Withania somnifera* or winter cherry): It balances vata and kapha dosha, is a proven nerve tonic and alleviates stress and anxiety. It improves brain function, sleep quality and memory. It also boosts testosterone and counters sexual debility. It is recommended for sportspersons, as it counters muscle weakness and muscle fatigue. Ashwagandha is one of the most powerful herbs in the Ayurvedic pharmacopoeia and is also an effective *rasayana.*

2. Amla (*Phyllanthus emblica* or Indian gooseberry): Amla has the unique property of having five different rasas (sweet, sour, astringent, pungent, bitter) except that of salt. It is one of the best natural sources of vitamin C. It balances the three doshas. It is a rasayana, meaning it has anti-ageing, rejuvenating properties.

3. Yashtimadhu/Mulethi (*Glycyrrhiza glabra* or liquorice):
   Mulethi works by liquefying kapha dosha and so it is
   used for sore throat and coughs. It is also excellent for
   treating chronic respiratory and digestive disorders,
   especially acidity. It helps reduce stress, boosts immunity
   and controls cholesterol. Mulethi is a powerful rasayana,
   besides being useful in weight management.

4. Jatamansi (*Nardostachys jatamansi* or Indian spikenard):
   This herb derives its name from the root words '*jata*'
   meaning hair and '*manasi*' meaning mind, and likewise
   is beneficial for the mind and hair. A powerful memory
   enhancer and nerve tonic, it is used to treat neurological
   disorders, such as epilepsy, insomnia, hysteria, convulsions,
   depression and mental weakness. It is also good for hair
   growth and skin.

5. Arjun (*Terminalia arjuna*): The bark of this plant helps
   in controlling cholesterol and hyperlipidaemia, thereby
   strengthening the heart.

6. Neem (*Azadirachta indica* or margosa): Ayurveda
   recommends neem for a range of ailments. It has
   antiviral, anti-cancer, antibacterial, anti-allergic and
   immunomodulatory properties. It is effective in treating
   a range of skin ailments and is useful in detoxing by
   purifying the blood.

7. Punarnawa (*Boerhavia diffusa* or spreading hogweed):
   This herb is useful for treating oedema wherever it may
   be in the body. It is a good diuretic, helping rejuvenate
   the kidneys. It is also used in treating anaemia and liver
   diseases and is an effective rasayana.

8. Giloy/guduchi/amrita (*Tinospora cordifolia* or heart-leaved moonseed): Described as the 'plant of immortality', giloy is a powerful immune modulator and a rasayana. It detoxes the blood and liver. It pacifies an aggravated pitta and is prescribed for managing fevers.

9. Senai (*Cassia angustifolia* or Indian senna): This herb is primarily used as a natural laxative.

10. Shankhpushpi (*Convolvulus prostratus* or morning glory): This flowering plant is a memory booster and aids concentration. It balances all the three doshas.

11. Shatavri (*Asparagus racemosus* or asparagus): This herb is known to promote physical stamina and immunity. It regulates oestrogen and is specifically prescribed for lactating mothers to increase the flow of milk. It is effective in balancing hormones in menopausal women. In men, it improves sexual health. In addition, it is a diuretic and aids digestion.

12. Pudina (*Mentha spicata* or mint): Pudina is a natural carminative that soothes the digestive system, calming all kinds of intestinal inflammation. It also clears a range of respiratory problems, such as lung congestion. It is often used in oral care because of its fresh fragrance and cleansing properties.

13. Ghritkumari (aloe vera): This household favourite is known for balancing the kapha and pitta doshas. Effective in treating burns and injuries, it has many benefits for the skin, which is why it is an ingredient in many skincare formulations. Aloe vera is an effective liver tonic, is good for the stomach and contains phytonutrients.

14. Sarpgandha (*Auvolfia serpentina* or Indian snakeroot): This medicinal plant relaxes the blood vessels and regulates nerve function in the vessels leading to the heart. Hence, it is widely used in the treatment of high blood pressure, hypertension, panic attacks, insomnia and asthma.

15. Surabhini Nimba (*Murraya koenigii*, curry leaves or meethi neem): A popular flavouring agent in most Indian and Sri Lankan cuisines, this plant is extremely beneficial for many digestive problems. It has anti-inflammatory, antimicrobial and anti-carcinogenic properties and is filled with a range of valuable micronutrients.

16. Bhutrina (*Cybopogon citratus* or lemongrass): Lemongrass is an effective *ampachana* or a toxin digester. It has anti-fungal and anti-inflammatory properties. Lemongrass essential oil purifies and heals and is used for treating acne and wounds.

17. Guggulu (*Commiphora mukul* or myrrh): Guggul is a black resin which is a nervine tonic, an aphrodisiac, a diuretic, burns ama, reduces cholesterol and is a powerful anti-inflammatory agent. It is one of the best rasayanas.

18. Bala (*Sidia cordifolia* or country mallow): Bala, which literally translates as 'strength', is a powerful rasayana that helps build muscle tissue and addresses all kinds of nerve disorders. It has astringent, emollient and aphrodisiacal properties.

19. Bhringhraj (*Eclipta prostrata* or false daisy): Bhringhraj rejuvenates the liver and is an excellent tonic to promote hair growth and texture.

20. *Haritaki* (Terminalia chebula): The name literally translates as 'remover of disease'. This versatile herb is a rasayana, i.e., has rejuvenating properties. It is an aphrodisiac, a carminative and a purgative and supports cardiac health.

21. Kutki (*Picrorhyza kurrua* or yellow gentian): Kutki is excellent for liver health. It is a powerful blood purifier that clears alcohol toxicity, reduces cholesterol and cleanses the alimentary tract. It has antioxidant and anti-inflammatory properties.

22. Tulsi (*Ocimum tenuiflorum* or holy basil): The tulsi plant is ubiquitous in all traditional Hindu households where it is worshipped daily. Tulsi has many therapeutic and antioxidant properties and is recommended for respiratory and digestive conditions. Some studies indicate that it has anti-carcinogenic and immunomodulating properties.

23. Brahmi (*Bacopa monnieri* or water hyssop): Described as the 'herb of grace', brahmi is an excellent brain tonic, energizing the nerves, intelligence and memory. It helps combat depression and enhance awareness and has been used for treating Alzheimer's disease. It is a powerful rasayana.

24. Pippali (*Piper longum* or Indian long pepper): Pippali is an effective expectorant and bronchodilator and is prescribed for colds and congestion. Pippali activates agni and is excellent for improving sperm motility, reducing obesity and improving heart and liver health.

Dashamool, which translates to 'ten roots', is one of the most powerful Ayurvedic formulations. It is made from the dried and powdered roots of five shrubs *(laghu panchmool)* and five trees *(vrihat panchmool)*. While each of these can be independently used for treating different ailments, together they are a potent blend with enormous benefits for the digestive, nervous and respiratory systems. It is commonly used as a herbal supplement to balance the doshas, improve immunity, build core strength and boost overall health.

The ten ingredients are:

Bilva (*Aegle marmelos* or Indian bael)

Agnimantha (*Premna integrifolia* or headache tree)

Kashmari (*Gmelina arborea* or beechwood)

Shyonaka (*Oroxylum indicum* or broken bones tree)

Patala (*Stereospermum suaveolens* or trumpet flower tree)

Sariva (*Hemedesmus indicus*)

Kantakari *(Solanum xanthocarpum* or yellow fruit nightshade)

Shalaparni (*Desmodium gangeticum*)

Prishniparni (*Uraria picta*)

Gokhru (*Tribulus terrestris*)

The *Charaka Samhita* cites shilajit as being one of the most interesting medicines in the Ayurveda pharmacopeia. It is a sticky resin-like mineral of plant origin, exuded from rocks found at high Himalayan altitudes. The Himalayas were formed due to the collision of the Indian plate and the Eurasian plate, a process that began 50 million years ago and still continues. When this tectonic shift happened, the forests were crushed between the rocks for millions of years. When temperatures are high, this herbo-mineral oozes out from cracks in the rock in the form of a nutrient-rich bitumen, which in Ayurveda is known as shilajit. The word shilajit derives from the root words '*shila*', meaning 'rock', and '*jit*', meaning 'victory'. Shilajit imparts rock-like strength and victory over the body. It is a rare and valuable rasayana which is sought after for its powerful aphrodisiacal and rejuvenating properties.

11

Deep Cleansing Within

Toxins are harmful substances that accumulate in the human system as a by-product of metabolic activities, environmental pollution, medication, faulty eating habits and unhealthy lifestyles. Over time, these toxins build up and begin to cause symptoms, such as oedema, poor circulation, anxiety, depression, weight gain, brain fog, gout, digestive disorders, insomnia, gas, sinus and respiratory issues, arthritis, fatigue and more. Free radicals are toxins in our environment that are highly reactive and can set off large chain reactions in our body, causing a range of damaging effects from premature ageing to cardiovascular diseases and cancer.

Toxins build up due to stress and negative mental attitudes. Conversely, they are also the cause of depression and negativity, in a vicious Catch-22 cycle. Ayurveda recognizes that toxicity is the cause of a host of ailments, and therefore, detox therapies constitute a huge component of its treatments. Apart from these dedicated detox therapies, most Ayurvedic drugs themselves have components that detox/cleanse the body. The human system has its own natural way of detoxing and cleansing the body through the excretory system. Apart from the obvious ways of waste removal through defecation and urination, the skin too excretes toxins through the sweat glands. The liver helps excrete hormones, drugs and other substances, while the lungs expel carbon dioxide from the blood. The whole human body is an extraordinary detox system, flushing out toxins day and night and even when you sleep.

Yet, despite this, over time, we accumulate toxins which, if we are not careful, can overwhelm and overload our natural excretory systems and result in illness. Therefore, inner cleansing is a foundational pillar in the science of Ayurveda.

Detox through panchkarma

Panchkarma is one of the cornerstones of Ayurveda. It includes five primary cleansing actions and related pre- and post-panchkarma procedures. Panchkarma tends to be quite a rigorous process and must only be undertaken under clinical supervision. Panchkarma purifies the body from within and without, clearing toxins and speeding up the metabolism by increasing agni. It unblocks the *srotas* or energy channels, relaxing and rejuvenating the body and mind and boosting immunity. While panchkarma is recommended in the treatment of particular ailments, it is also recommended that healthy individuals undergo panchkarma about thrice a year in order to maintain their vitality. Panchkarma is best

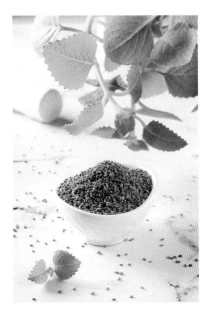

Ajwain seeds and plant

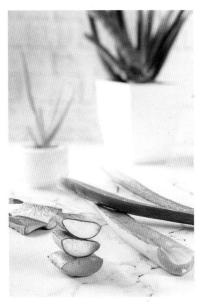

Aloe Vera gel and plant

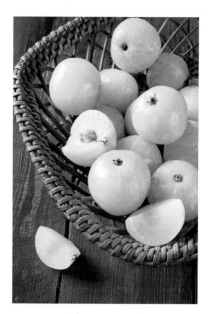

Amla (Indian Gooseberry)

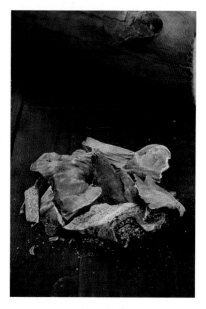

Arjun bark

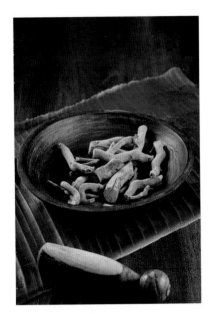

Ashwagandha root

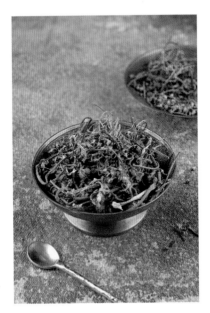

Bahringraj

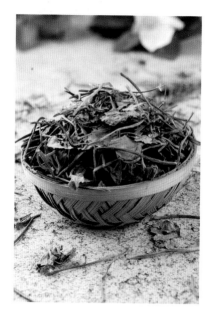

Brahmi

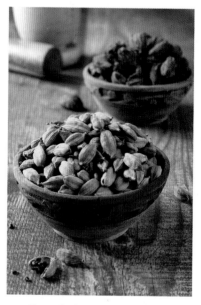

Chotti, badi elaichi (Cardamom)

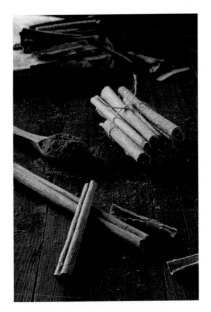

Cinnamon sticks and powder

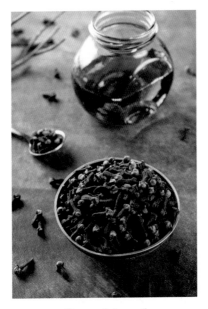

Clove and clove oil

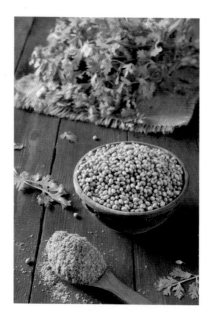

Coriander leaves, seeds and powder

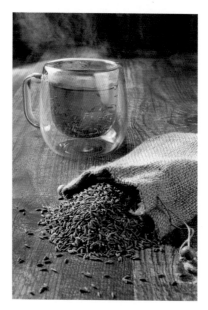

Cumin and Cumin water

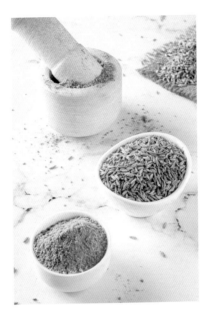

Fennel seeds and fennel powder

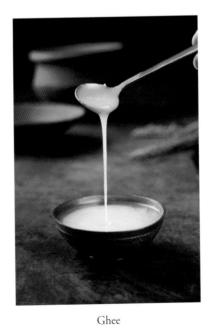

Ghee

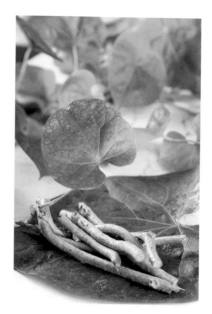

Giloy

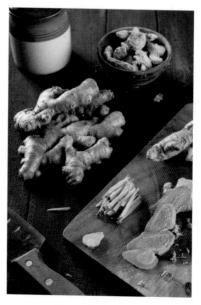

Ginger fresh and dry

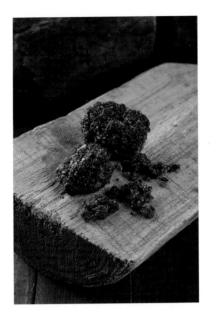

Guggulu

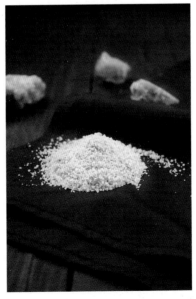

Hing (Asafoetida)

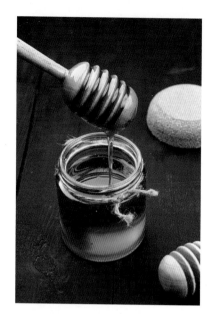

Honey

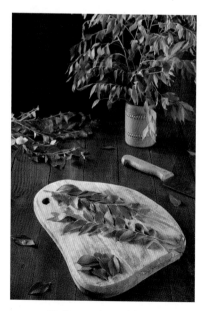

Kadi patta (curry leaves)

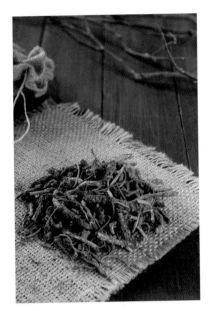

Kutaki

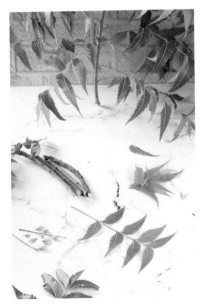

Neem branches, leaves and Nimoli

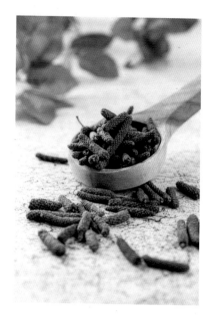

Peepli

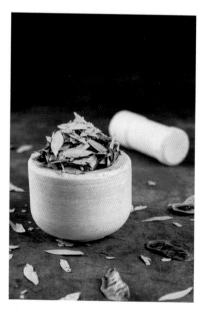

Sanai patti

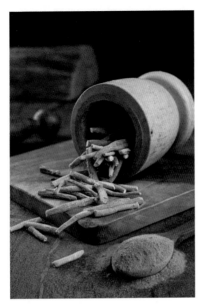

Sarpgandha root and powder

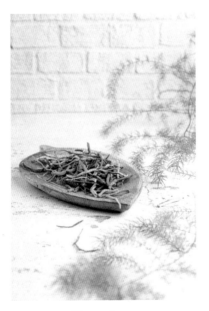

Shatavari root

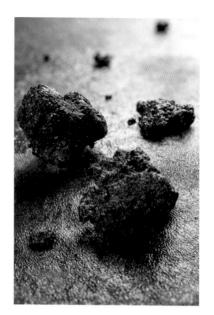

Shilajit

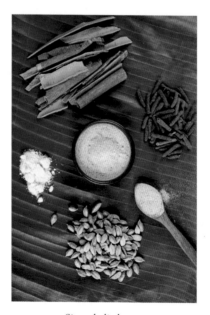

Sitopaladi churna

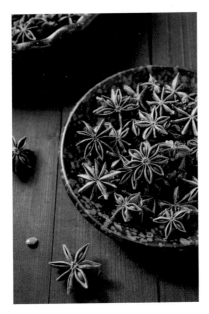

Star anise

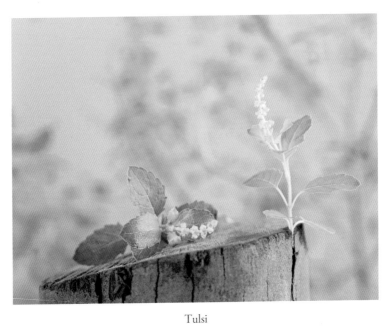

Tulsi

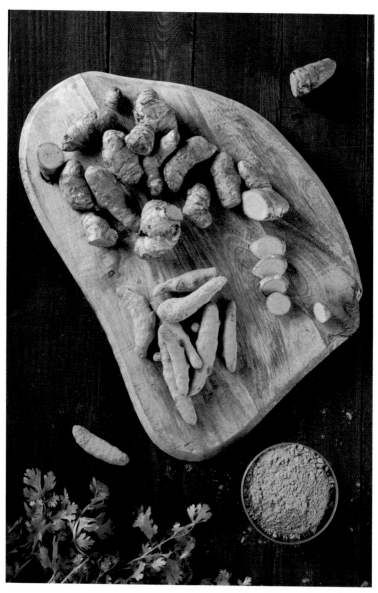

Turmeric fresh, dried and powder

taken during *ritusandhikaal*, i.e., the juncture of the seasons in June-July, March-April and October-November. While a full Panchkarma involves five processes, each one of these is a full treatment in itself.

Panchkarma involves five distinct procedures:

1. *Vamana* is the first step. It involves abhyanga or massaging the body with warm medicinal oils. The patient is also given emetic preparations to induce vomiting and remove toxins. This is followed up by hot fomentation or steaming with medicinal herbs to induce a sweat. Toxins in the body are loosened by the medicinal oils and can then be flushed out through fomentation. Vamana by itself is often prescribed for kapha-related conditions.

2. *Virechan* is the second step. The previous step of vamana helps push the ama or toxins into the small intestine. In this step, together with oil massage and herbal steam, the patient is given natural purgatives to clear the toxins out of the alimentary canal. Virechan alone is commonly prescribed for pitta-related ailments.

3. *Basti* is the third step. This step involves administering enemas to clean and heal the gut. Enemas could be of ghee, medicinal oils, milk or herbal decoctions depending on the condition to be addressed. Basti alone is prescribed for many vata-related conditions.

4. *Nasya* is the fourth step. While the earlier steps focused on the body neck downwards, nasya addresses the head. After a preparatory massage and steam inhalation, nasal drops, which could be medicinal oils or herbal decoctions,

are administered. This cleanses the sinuses and addresses various kinds of congestion in the face and head area. *Shirodhara, shirobasti* and *netratarpan* are other therapies that address issues related to the head.

5. *Raktamokshan* is the final step. This treatment involves bloodletting to cleanse the blood of impurities and toxic material. Traditionally, leeches were used for this purpose. In fact, in the iconography of Lord Dhanvantri, the deity of the science of Ayurveda is depicted holding a leech in his hand. Nowadays, bloodletting is done with medical syringes.

Apart from curing physical ailments through the deep tissue detox that panchkarma offers, the treatment delivers great emotional and psychological benefits. Emotions such as fear, anxiety, grief and anger in the form of neurotransmitters become locked into the body tissues. The massaging of medicated oils in abhyanga and fomentation with herbal infusions help to release blocked emotions by stimulating the blocked neurotransmitters. Detox in Ayurveda is as much a purification of the mind as of the body.

Detox through fasting

'Langhanam param aushadham'—*Ashtanghridayam*
('Fasting is the highest medicine')

Fasting is common to almost all religious traditions as it is universally held to yield great spiritual benefits. Meditation is usually prescribed along with fasting. The principle is simple. The body is energy and if we do not expend that energy on metabolic activity, that energy can be channelled upwards towards spiritual growth. When we fast, the body feels lighter and is more conducive to higher goals.

Ayurveda prescribes fasting as a simple means of detox that we can all practise as part of our routine. Fasting allows the digestive system to rest and recoup. When the body is given a break from the daily onslaught of the toxins we eat, it has an opportunity to break down and eliminate accumulated toxins. Fasting also stimulates a process called autophagy, in which cells recycle and renew their content. Yoshinori Ohsumi, a Japanese biologist and Nobel Laureate, in his ground-breaking research on autophagy, describes this process and how it results in cell renewal and longevity.[15] Ayurveda has always recognized fasting as a means to cell renewal.

Fasting as a cure for illness is a phenomenon that is actually built into the natural intelligence of the body. We have observed how birds and animals instinctively stop eating when they are sick. When we are sick, the body needs to direct all its energies towards resisting the illness instead of using it to digest food. If food is taken while we are sick, our energies are wasted on digestion. So the body, in its wisdom, naturally reduces our appetite and we do not feel like eating. What happens next is even more interesting. The body needs to generate heat energy, and in the absence of food, it begins to burn stored toxins that are, in fact, the cause of our illness. In this way, a self-healing process takes place. The well-known nineteenth-century physician Dr Edward Dewey wrote, 'When a patient stops taking food, it is the disease and not the patient that dies of starvation.' We do not need to wait to fall sick in order to fast. Whenever we fast, the body will begin to burn and eliminate toxins.

Fasting is called *langhana* in Ayurveda, which derives from the root word '*laghu*' which means 'light'. *Langhana* could be either *anshana* or a full fast, or it could be *laghuanshana*, which is partaking of only light food. Anshana is only prescribed during high fever, diarrhoea, vomiting and other such extreme conditions. For the purposes of detox, Ayurveda does not recommend anshana but prefers a mono-diet of single, easily digestible food.

Khichri, a light gruel of dhuli moong dal (husked green gram) and rice, is one of the best foods for fasting and suits all body types. The gruel should be seasoned with cumin and asafoetida roasted in ghee.

For vata-dominant people, a fasting diet of rice and toor/arhar dal (yellow split pigeon peas) is best. A pitta person should have dhuli moong dal (husked green gram) and rice, while a millet porridge is best for kapha-dominant people.

Fruit and juice fasts are recommended only for people with strong constitutions and no pathological disorders. Dr Vasant Lad recommends that a juice fast not be undertaken more than once every few months. He suggests that vata types can drink the juice of sweet oranges, mangoes or grapes. For pitta types, sweet grapes, cranberry and pomegranate juice are recommended. Kapha types can choose apple, grape and pineapple juice.

Ayurveda does not recommend prolonged fasting as that reduces the agni in the body. It is best to fast about twice a week as a simple detox routine. It is also particularly important to keep yourself well-hydrated during these fasts. It is also very important to ease yourself slowly into your normal diet, gradually increasing your intake and food items.

Detox in daily life

Ayurveda has been designed as not only a field of medicine but as a way of life. Simple methods of detoxing the body can be built into our everyday life. One of the most common practices is that of a weekly purge using herbal preparations, such as triphala. Triphala, which is a combination of three medicinal fruits, is taken with warm water to purge the alimentary canal and flush out toxins. Another good purgative is 1.5 to 2 teaspoons of castor oil taken with lukewarm water at bedtime.

Other methods include drinking a glass of boiled and lukewarm barley water. This works as an effective diuretic. A couple of teaspoons of Indian gooseberry juice or a single gooseberry boiled in water is an excellent detox remedy. It is advisable that the raw amla juice should not come into contact with any metal. The pulp/juice of aloe vera also has wonderful detox properties.

All of these are simple home remedies to cleanse your body on an ongoing basis and prevent a build-up of toxins that will otherwise certainly lead to disease. A clean gut is the key to health and these simple everyday detoxes are the secret to a healthy digestion and a glowing complexion.

12

Drinking from the Fountain of Youth

The American civil rights activist Frances Lear famously said that she believed that the second half of one's life was meant to be better than the first.[16] The first half is to find out how to do things correctly in life and the second half is to enjoy doing it the right way. Right knowledge paves the way to living youthfully even in the second part of life.

Fortunately, Ayurveda devotes a whole field of its knowledge to resisting the depredations of time on mind and body. The market is flooded with anti-ageing solutions for skin and hair but these remain superficial and temporary. Likewise, surgical interventions that promise a youthful face and body often result in a grotesque and unnatural appearance, especially in those who are old and mature. Neither surgery nor chemical products address the fundamental problems of ageing.

Agni, the fire of youth

Youth lies within and the secret to looking and feeling young lies in our agni dosha—the very fire of our life. In Ayurveda, it is said, 'A person is as old as his or her agni.' Agni is the real doorway to youthfulness. Our immune system is healthy when our agni is strong. A person whose metabolic fires are strong can expect to live a long, healthy and youthful life. If we consider God to be pure awareness, agni should be revered as the mouth of that pure awareness. Awareness is the bridge between the lower and higher consciousness and agni is the doorway to that awareness, the bridge between the lower self and the purer/divine self. Agni governs the destruction of old cells and the creation of the new ones.

Breathing holds the key

'He who binds the breath, binds the mind. He who binds the mind, binds the breath.'—*Hatha Yoga Pradipika*

Each cell in our body is alive and breathing. Breathing is of two kinds: aerobic and anaerobic. For aerobic breathing, oxygen is necessary as this is connected to prana vayu, which speeds up oxidation and ageing. Aerobic breathing maintains metabolism and oxidation and burns up the free radicals. On the other hand, while performing different types of pranayamas, the attempt is to increase the anaerobic component of breathing. Anaerobic breath utilizes carbon dioxide to enhance the life of our cells. Anaerobic breathing is connected to apana vayu or the anchoring breath, which increases the life span of each cell. All forms of pranayama relate to retention of breath or reducing aerobic breathing. According to Ayurveda, our longevity depends on our breathing rate—more accurately, the rate at which we inhale. The giant tortoise with a breathing rate of four breaths/ minute lives up to 200 years. Among humans, the slower and deeper our breaths, the healthier our cells and the longer our lifespan. Simply put, the slower you breathe, the longer you will live. Pranayamas that prescribe short, quick breaths focus on swift and sharp exhalations, thereby limiting the aerobic component and increasing the anaerobic component of breathing.

Our body can live and sustain itself on a limited amount of oxygen. The best example of this are yogis who live for more than a hundred years doing yoga and pranayama exercises. Pranayama slows the process of ageing as anaerobic breathing becomes proactive. When we are in a deep meditative state, our breathing slows to the minimum possible pace, causing body cells to perform anaerobic breathing. When we sleep, our breath slows. This contributes to longevity. During sleep, the body produces hormones that contribute to youthful appearance, energy and strength. What we essentially need to note is that the faster we breathe, the faster our metabolism works and the faster we age. On the other hand, slowing down our breathing also slows down our metabolism and thus enhances the span of the cellular life.

Thinking young

'We are what we think. All that we are arises from our thoughts. With our thoughts we make the world.'—
Gautama Buddha

Every cell contains within itself intelligence and memory. Hence, together with breathing, our thoughts, whether conscious or subconscious, contribute to ageing. It is often said that thoughts become actions and we become what we think. That's because thoughts are the most powerful electromagnetic pulse forms of energy that affect not just our body but even our root connection with consciousness itself. In our daily experience, thoughts manifest as a powerful tool for either our well-being or for our destruction. Every thought produces corresponding emotions, which then cause biochemical changes in our blood and plasma. The state of our rasa dhatu (plasma) is a good mirror of this phenomenon. If, through our thoughts, we positively influence the quality of our plasma, it becomes possible to live a long and youthful life. Ayurveda advises us to develop a consciously positive attitude towards life and living in order to rejuvenate our rasa dhatu and pave the way to longevity.

Effect of doshas on ageing

The three doshas play a vital role in longevity and in maintaining cellular health. People who are predominantly pitta type tend to look mature while vata types look distinctly older. Kapha types are the fortunate ones who tend to look young. Besides its other important functions, kapha is also responsible for building new cells, which is why people of this type are able to maintain a youthful look. The deterioration and degeneration of our body takes place at the cellular level, and therefore, rejuvenation also takes place at this level.

Vata skin is dry, thin, fine-pored and cool to the touch. It tends to develop wrinkles fairly early. Pitta skin is fair, soft and warm to the touch. It has least tolerance to sun and is most likely to suffer damage due to exposure to the sun. Kapha skin is thick, oily, soft and cool to touch and tends to develop wrinkles much later in life than the others.

As explained earlier, each dosha's function is to support and sustain the functions of billions of cells in the human body. The proper stability of the doshas produces one's aura, which is our defence shield, protecting us from harmful intrusions. Ojas is the substance of our aura, tejas gives the aura its colour and prana is the movement of the aura. The stronger one's aura, the happier and relatively younger one stays.

Remaining robust with rasayanas

We have learned that agni, cellular breathing, the three doshas and our aura together are the factors that determine our physical and mental state. Ayurveda recommends rejuvenation therapies based on the science of rasayanas. Rasayanas are elixirs or herbal medicines that delay ageing and prolong life. Consuming rasayanas is an effective way to enhance our agni, balance our doshas and maintain our dhatus and ojas. This will counter and minimize the effects of ageing. Unlike modern supplements, rasayanas literally enter the rasa dhatu (plasma) to enhance our agni energy. Ayurveda aims at maintaining the health of a healthy person and curing the disease of an unhealthy one. The functional power of a rasayana is quite astonishing because it gives positive results in both cases. It increases health and eradicates diseases. The word 'rasayana' is made up of rasa, which means taste as well as plasma, and *ayana*, meaning 'to enter'. Though Ayurvedic rasayanas can be specific to certain tissues and channels, they can also be used to rejuvenate all bodily tissues. They also promote health and healing by helping to balance the three doshas, the seven dhatus and the three malas. Further, the rasayanas bring about balance between prana, tejas and ojas. Rasayanas are 'the kings of health and healing'.

Common single-herb rasayanas

Herbal medicines are prescribed according to the dhatus they affect and as per the dosha constitution of the person. Some of the powerful herbs which are used as rasayanas are:

Amalki, ashwagandha, guggulu, haritaki (harad), shatavri, guduchi (giloy), punarnava and pippali. These have the following qualities of *dipana* (increases agni), *pachana* (burns toxins), *balya* (gives strength), *jivaniya* (supports life) and *bruhana* (provides nutrition).

Vata type people are advised to take ashwagandha or guggulu or dashamool rasayana. Pitta type people should go for shatavri or guduchi rasayana. Kapha-dominant people should choose pippali or punarnava rasayana to increase agni.

Seasons too need to be taken into consideration. In the early spring and winter, one should have a rasayana that is warm in nature, like pippali rasayana. As spring gives way to summer, one should switch over to shatavri rasayana because it is calming and cooling. For fall and approaching winter, ashwagandha rasayana, which pacifies vata, is ideal.

Aushadha rasayanas

Aushadha rasayanas refer to medicinal formulations or compounds. Chyawanprash is one of the most popular and commonly used aushadha rasayans.

It is best to have one teaspoon of chyawanprash, preferably every morning and evening in the winters, and half a teaspoon of chyawanprash every morning and evening in the summers. Avoid having water for half an hour after consuming chyawanprash.

It is said that the recipe for Brahm Rasayana came from Lord Brahma himself and is a powerful anti-ageing formula. Dashamool rasayan is another powerful tonic that is used for a range of conditions.

Ashwagandha *churna* and triphala powder are potent aushadha rasayanas. Triphala powder is best had mixed with ghee and jaggery. For best absorption, ashwagandha should be had with warm milk. Other alternatives are with honey or lukewarm water. The choice of aushadha rasayana will vary according to season, a person's prakruti (constitution) and *vikruti* (imbalance).

While the term rasayana generally refers to tonics and herbal preparations (aushadha rasayana*)*, the field of *rasayana chikitsa* is much broader in scope. The other important rasayanas are:

Atma rasayana (pertaining to the mind), *ahara rasayana* (diet), *vihara rasayana* (lifestyle) and *achara-vichara rasayana* (behaviour)

(1) Atma rasayana comes first. It simply means that we feed our minds with pure, positive thoughts. This is the best way for self-rejuvenation. The more we think positive and think 'young', the more we will inculcate the feeling of youthfulness. This feeling itself, if sustained as a discipline, will induce physiological changes in our bodies.

(2) Ahara rasayana: This refers to the diet suited to one's constitution. The correct diet will correct the aggravated dosha while balancing the other two doshas, and will also support the dhatus. The following is suggested:

For vata dosha: 3–5 soaked almonds daily, 4–5 soaked anjeer (figs), 5 large soaked raisins and 2 full walnuts. The almonds should only be taken during the monsoon and winter.

For pitta dosha: Have a bowl of rice pudding with 2–3 small cardamoms daily. Also, 2–4 soaked almonds, 4–5 soaked anjeer (figs), 5 large soaked raisins and 2 full walnuts. The almonds should be consumed only during the monsoons and winter by the pitta type.

For kapha dosha: Take 5–8 soaked almonds, 2–4 walnuts, 4–5 soaked anjeer and a similar amount of raisins throughout the year.

Cashews should be had very sparingly by all types, and especially those with kapha dosha, as they are high in cholesterol and fats. All the dry fruits should first be washed thoroughly before soaking. It is recommended that you drink the water in which the anjeer and raisins have been soaked.

(3) Vihara rasayana: This means following a lifestyle and routine specifically suited to our dosha configuration. This includes our waking and sleep time, our work hours, meal timings, exercise regime, recreation etc.

For vata dosha: Have an oil massage daily. Also, bathe in water infused with ginger extract and a pinch of baking soda. Take care to keep yourself sufficiently warm in the winters. Rub slightly warm sesame and coconut oil (if it's comfortable) on the scalp and the soles of the feet at bedtime. Observe celibacy for considerable periods. A brief afternoon siesta is recommended.

For pitta dosha: In summers, take a cold bath, apply sandalwood paste on your forehead and apply freshly crushed henna (mehendi) leaves on the soles of your feet. Try to stay in the shade and use shades in the sun. A brief afternoon siesta is recommended.

For kapha dosha: Take a daily massage with warm mustard oil. Practise yoga. Go for dynamic exercises. Take hot showers. Sleeping during the daytime in the winters or monsoons is not recommended.

(4) Achara-vichara rasayana: Ayurveda holds that there is inherent healing power in a person's own positive behaviour. When a person meditates and lives in harmony within themselves, when they live in harmony with the ecology and with those around them and live ethically and with a clear conscience, it affects the way their physiology functions. Following the prescriptions of this form of rasayana, a person can keep their faculties and body youthful and healthful.

13

Ayurveda and Beauty

From hair loss to hair growth

Everyone is the king or queen of their own life and one's hair is their crowning glory. Though we may like to believe that our real glory lies in our happy mind, we cannot deny that having a good head of hair matters a lot to us. For almost all of us, lush hair boosts our confidence and courage. Obviously, it all starts from the top.

While the market is filled with a plethora of products that promise to reduce hair fall, thicken growth or improve texture, it is advisable not to fall for quick-fix solutions. Ayurveda educates us on facts about hair and skin that television advertisements do not tell us. In the human body, hair and nails are biological tools that serve as exit routes for things that need to be removed from the body. Hair and nails are the exit points of *asthi vaha srotas* or the channels that carry nutrition to the bone tissues through the skeletal system. Our body constantly eliminates unwanted toxic molecules, excreting them through the asthi vaha srotas. This process helps the body maintain its water-electrolyte balance. Hair has no nerve endings, and so we feel no sensation when it is cut. But if our hair is pulled or nails are cut close to the skin, we feel the pain. This is because majja dhatu (muscle) is present at the root of hair and nails. Since asthi dhatu or bone tissue is excreted through the nails, these serve as an indicator of the condition of our asthi dhatu. The quality of the asthi dhatu is mirrored in the quality of the nails. Brittle nails mean brittle asthi dhatu and vice versa. When we start losing hair or if our nails turn brittle, it is a clear indication that the bones are becoming brittle and this condition needs to be treated.

Let us now understand the reasons that lead to hair fall. There is a tiny opening near the root of each hair, which is connected to the sweat gland. Sweat, by virtue of it being an oily substance, strengthens the root of the hair. But if this sebaceous secretion is in excess, the hair loses its grip and falls off. This is the simple reason behind hair fall. The glow and lustre of hair is attributed to the power of pitta, which creates heat in the body. The word pitta is a derivative of the Sanskrit word 'tapa', which means 'to become hot'. However, the excess heating up of the body produces excessive sweat, which in turn can lead to hair loss. Other causes of hair loss are hormonal imbalances, dandruff, chemical treatments, illness, inadequate nutrition, side-effects of medicines or even tying the hair too tightly.

Ayurvedic tips for hair growth

The scalp should be kept clean if one wants lustrous and thick hair. It is advised to massage the scalp using Mahabhringhraj oil and not the one with just the essence in it.

A head massage is suggested thrice a week with coconut oil, warm olive oil or mustard oil.

Massaging curd on the scalp and leaving it for 15–20 minutes before shampooing once a week helps in cleaning the scalp and nourishing the hair roots.

Massage the scalp with fresh amla juice or amla powder soaked in water, once in ten days. This should be left for at least 20–30 minutes before shampooing.

Crushed fresh henna (mehendi) mixed with any oil should be massaged on the scalp once every fortnight for lustrous hair.

For maintaining hair colour: Boil half a teaspoon of tea leaves in half a litre of water and use the liquid to do the final rinse after shampooing. Once in a fortnight will suffice.

Apply equal quantities of amla and shikakai powder to the scalp and do a massage once a month, to maintain hair health. After application, this mixture should be left for approximately 10–15 minutes prior to shampooing.

From dry, rough skin to smooth, soft skin

Emotions play an important part in the condition of our skin. Stress causes stress lines to appear on our forehead and being constantly worried robs the face of its glow. When we are angry, our facial skin appears hot and flushed, and when we are joyful, the skin on our face acquires a lustre. Beneath the epidermis is a layer of a connective tissue within which are accumulated biochemical impulses of anger, fear, stress, unresolved issues, etc. The outer layer or epidermis responds to and reflects these emotions, whether positive or negative. The connection between emotions and the response of it on our skin is made and navigated by prana. What this means is that our skin is constantly 'breathing prana' and thereby reflecting our deepest emotions, both conscious and unconscious.

Ayurveda holds that radiant skin and beauty are direct results of good mental and physical health. In terms of the doshas, components of the three kinds of pitta have to work in tandem to maintain skin health. *Bhrajaka pitta*, a sub-type of pitta, brings brightness to the skin; *ranjika pitta* gives colour, lustre and glow and *pachaka pitta* helps digestion. A glowing skin represents a state of balanced pitta. The skin is also connected to all the internal organs. If rakta dhatu is too high, the cheeks become flushed. If rakta dhatu is low, the skin becomes pallid, dull, dry and cracked.

Ayurveda holds that it is important to have a moderate amount of fat in order to have a firm skin. This may vary as per the structure and weight of the body. Whether the quality or quantity of fat is in correct measure for a particular individual is revealed by their pulse.

There are seven layers of skin. Each layer is designed to support the layer above it. The outermost layer is connected to the rasa dhatu (nutrient fluid, plasma). This is reflected in a person's aura and is a mirror of their health. The second layer relates to the rakta dhatu. The third layer is connected to mamsa dhatu (muscle) and contributes to skin colour. Any impurities in the inner layers will show up in the outermost layer. Excluding the two topmost layers, the inner layers are referred to as *up-dhatus* of mamsa. The fourth layer aids the immune system and prevents skin infections. The fifth layer reflects the association of the skin with the rest of the body. It is due to this that one feels different sensations. The sixth layer helps in the healing and regeneration of one's system. The seventh layer acts as a base for the other layers and contributes to the skin's firmness. The health of these different layers determines the quality and glow of a person's skin.

Ayurveda for good skin

Good skin is not just about having good looks. It has immense contribution in removing the impurities from the plasma. If our skin is wrinkling too fast, it means that our rasa dhatu could be in an inferior state. In such cases, instead of applying lotions on our skin, it would be better if we found solutions to improve our rasa dhatu with the help of an Ayurvedic physician. It should be understood that our body sweat is an oily liquid, which keeps our skin soft and moist. Hence, it is of immense value in the contribution of removing the impurities from the plasma. Clean skin facilitates our sweat glands in secreting perspiration in the correct manner beneficial to us.

Skin is always exposed to air. Accordingly, the skin should be protected from too much heat, chemical pollution etc. It should never be overexposed to the sun or to air that has too much dust or pollution.

Purifying our blood via Ayurvedic formulations from time to time is very important for healthy skin. Hence, for that purpose, the use of *maha manjisht adyarisht, anant salsa* syrup, *sari vadhyarisht, rakta shodhak bhati, khadirarisht, chopyachiniyadi churna* etc. are suggested under expert supervision.

For clear and smooth skin, women should have regular periods. If the bleeding is inadequate, then *rajah pravarthini bati* is advised and to regularize the cycle of menstruation, *ashokarisht* and *sundari kalp* are beneficial. Again, this has to be taken under expert supervision.

Some tips for maintaining healthy skin

(i) Consume two to three full teaspoons of cow's ghee daily.

(ii) Avoid overuse of salt as it is not good for the skin and can cause eczema and dermatitis.

(iii) Avoid overuse of sour food as it can cause skin rashes and acne.

(iv) Hydration and massage are of utmost importance to keep our skin suitably hydrated. You can do this by having eight to ten glasses of water every day. Massaging with the right strokes using natural oils as per our constitution is highly recommended.

(v)   Applying and massaging with almond oil is good for the facial skin.

(vi)   Application of coconut oil or mustard oil on the face at regular intervals is a must. If there's any infection on the skin, neem oil can also be used sparingly.

(vii) To have pure blood running under the facial epidermis, have a guava or a pomegranate every day.

(viii) Chewing three to five small tender neem leaves every alternate day ensures infection-free skin.

(ix)   Skin has to be moisturized often. Using good quality sunscreen throughout the year in the daytime protects the skin from the UV rays and dust. It is of utmost importance to remember that facial skin should not be exposed to the sun for a long time.

(x)   When the air is polluted, use a herbal sunscreen at night, to protect the facial skin.

(xi)   Consumption of triphala powder mixed with lukewarm water is very good for balancing the three doshas. Having it daily maintains the quality of the skin and hair.

(xii) In case of severe itching on skin, mix 20–30 grams of pure camphor powder in half a litre of coconut oil and massage.

(xiii) Oil pulling is advised for maintaining contours of the facial muscles. Use one tablespoon of coconut or sesame oil.

(xiv) Regular facial exercises help in keeping the face young. Contracting and expanding the mouth helps the facial muscles remain firm.

(xv) Expressions on the face have a strong impact in making us look youthful and smart. Joyful expressions and a calm demeanour can make us look charming. On the other hand, negative expressions like frowns, furrowed brows and pressed lips etc. can make us look grumpy and older.

Home-made Lotion

Take about fifteen to twenty petals of common Indian red rose, drop them in a bottle or a jar of a quarter litre olive oil and keep it in the sun every day for one to two hours. The fine qualities of both rose and olive will be blended naturally by solar power and heat. The bottle should be placed in the sun for one to two hours for about fifteen to twenty days consecutively to prepare our effective potion. Application of this enhances the glow of the face.

14

The Science of Stress

'Hridaye chetana sthanam'—*Charaka Samhita*
'The heart is the seat of consciousness.'

To achieve a state of emotional balance, there has to be harmony between one's thoughts and emotions. The link between the mind and heart is controlled by a sub-dosha of pitta dosha called sadhaka pitta. It enables us to digest and transform our external experiences into inner experiential wisdom. In anatomical terms, sadhaka pitta includes the neurotransmitters that help us mentally metabolize and make sense of our experiences.

'Cultivation of the mind is as necessary as food is to the body.'—Marcus Tullius Cicero

We tend not to take seriously that which is not visible. The mind is an invisible factor. The fact is that science has not yet arrived at any conclusion about what actually constitutes the mind, or even whether it is distinguishable from the brain. Hence, it is easily dismissible.

One can imagine the incredulous responses from people when Gautama Buddha said, 'The mind is everything; what you think you become.' Even twenty-four centuries later, many find it hard to believe that this invisible phenomenon can decide and dictate the very fate of their lives.

From the mind sprouts joy and misery, which are reflected in our body. Soma means body, psyche means mind. Put together, they become the term psychosomatic, which gives us a clue to Ayurveda's view of diseases as expressions of psychological disharmonies. All illnesses are symptoms of complex psychosomatic phenomena. Ayurveda teaches us that our state of mind is dependent on whichever guna or quality is predominant in our nature, whether satva, rajas or tamas. The conscious handling of the gunas is a powerful way of maintaining mental and emotional equilibrium.

Each individual contains within themselves the three gunas in varying degrees. When rajas is predominant, it gives rise to strong desires, ambition, competitiveness, anger, euphoria, anxiety and other strong feelings. What is very interesting about the attribute of rajas is that it has the capacity of tilting towards either tamas or satva. When tamas is dominant, we experience feelings of depression, dependency, addiction, apathy, grief, ignorance, guilt, shame etc. Tamas tends to cause the mind to close down on itself, alienating the person from their environment and slowing down their actions. Sattvic guna leads to feelings of empathy, equanimity, bliss, freedom, self-control and wellness. Satva is aligned with the unalterable cosmic laws and therefore harmonizes the external and internal aspects of a person. A conscious person can evolve to manage their gunas according to the demands of their environment, irrespective of which guna is naturally predominant within them.

The mystery of the mind–body connection

The play of the gunas demonstrate how the drama that takes place in our mind is reflected in our behaviour and even in our bodies. All *adharmas* (wrong thoughts and actions) in behaviour originate in the mind. Additionally, wrong thoughts affect the body, impairing the efficiency and balance of the doshas. Ayurveda has always emphasized the inter-relationship of the mind and the body in causing either illness or health.

There are enough clinical studies that prove that maladies like headaches, abdominal pain, digestion problems, anxiety, depression, BP, skin problems, heart attacks, strokes, insomnia etc. are linked to unmanaged anger/frustration that is bottled up within us. Tension, stress, strain, emotional instabilities and phobias also cause damage to our bodies. The metabolic changes caused by these afflictions can reduce the agni energy, which in turn leads to disease. Stress in the nervous system results in mandagni, which then inhibits the gastric secretions. At the same time, stress results in an over-stimulation of the sympathetic nervous system, causing an increase in the secretion of adrenaline.

Just because the mind-body connection remains invisible, we cannot ignore it. Once we find that this has a direct impact on us, there is no more mystery, and we can then work towards a holistic change in our mental make-up.

When it comes to psychosomatic conditions, there's a popular misconception that it is all in the 'head', and therefore there is a certain social stigma attached to it. Psychosomatic conditions are looked down upon, even by qualified doctors, as being 'mental issues'. Hence, people are afraid to express these openly and often effective treatments are not administered in time. Some also believe that these issues will somehow get resolved on their own. It is important to know that the physical symptoms of any psychosomatic condition are very real and require treatment, just like any other illnesses.

Signs and symptoms of stress

Mental stress manifests itself in different ways in different people. Spotting the signs and symptoms will help in diagnosis and also help determine the specific causes. Common physical signs of mental stress are palpitations, fast heart rate, increased perspiration, sweaty palms, panic attacks, fatigue despite getting enough rest and sleep, low libido or an increase in sex drive, tense muscles, chest pain, high BP, irritability or a tremble in the stomach often described as 'butterflies in the stomach'. In women, stress can also manifest as changes in the menstrual cycle and abdominal bloating.

Age groups most vulnerable

Stress symptoms vary depending on the age group. Children under stress could suffer from frequent stomach aches or skin rashes. Signs of nervousness may include rubbing their eyes or touching body parts. Stress is common among teenagers because at their age, they undergo dramatic hormonal changes. Moreover, during the teen years, there is heavy pressure due to parental expectations and demands for social adjustment, which could also lead to adolescent depression. At this age, children tend to become rebellious and may get addicted to drugs, alcohol or video games. In the elderly, stress appears as depression and even dementia since they are already facing compounding factors that affect their emotional well-being. While ageing by itself is a difficult process, it is compounded by the fact that elders often face rejection, abandonment, isolation, loss of vigour and chronic health problems.

Understanding stress

There are two ways to understand stress in the body. We can compare ourselves to a pressure cooker which, if the steam is vented, works very well. If not, pressure will build inside it until the lid blows. When it bursts, it bursts at its weakest point. This is how it is with human stress. If we cannot vent our emotions and keep suppressing them, we will reach bursting point and damage our health. The second analogy is of that of a river. If a river becomes flooded, it will ultimately overflow its banks. When the human mind is flooded with pent-up emotions, unexpressed negative thoughts and unrequited desires, a point is reached when these will break the dam of our control, leaving us 'broken' in some way. Both physical and psychological therapy is needed to fix these ruptures in the human system.

We do get warning signs or pointers prior to such stressful breakdowns. The 'ruptures' tend to manifest themselves around whichever body part in us is most vulnerable. If we have a weak digestion, then a stomach ache could be a stress symptom. Headaches could escalate into migraines due to stress. If our immunity is low, infections will take longer to heal.

Stress starts in the brain, causing a cascade of biochemical releases in the body, such as that of adrenaline, which triggers the primeval 'fight or flight' response. The body does not differentiate between physical threat and mental pain. If we are upset, the body will release the same hormones. If the body is exposed to a sustained release of cortisol and other stress hormones for a long time, our health will be impacted. Often, physicians address only the physical symptoms, ignoring the underlying mental causes. It is important for patients to receive both psychological therapies as well as pharmacological treatments.

Dealing with mental stress

It is recommended that we examine and identify memories, ideas and beliefs that do not serve our interests. It is important to accept and love ourselves as we are, granting our psyche permission to make allowances for our perceived shortcomings. We need to avoid self-pity and take responsibility/ownership of our life situations. We need to release ourselves from the pressure of social expectations. We need to identify areas of needless guilt in our mind and let go of the past. Forgiving ourselves is an immensely healing action. We need to release ourselves from the pressure of our own unrealistic goals. It is important to see our lives in perspective and not take life too seriously. All that we need to do is to make our best efforts in whichever direction we choose. There are simple mechanisms we can adopt to help us reach this state of being. These are:

i)   Being honest with yourselves and with others when seeking help. Accepting our state of mind or situation is the best way to zero in on the correct solution(s).

ii) Confiding in a well-meaning, trusted friend may put us on the path to positive recovery.

iii) Learning effective relaxation techniques, like watching humorous shows and stand-up comedy, listening to talks by trusted spiritual teachers, practising guided meditations and breathing exercises, playing with pets and engaging in relaxing hobby(ies) etc.

iv) Taking out time for enjoyable leisure activities that calm and relax us, such as music, dance, art etc.

v)   Joining a support group made up of like-minded people.

vi) Joking about stress, by making cartoons or telling humorous stories, thus enabling one to take the situation lightly.

vii) Taking a break to be close to nature. Nature has the power to heal at a very deep level. Taking regular breaks to connect with the outdoors helps bring down stress levels.

viii) Spending time in a new environment or culture takes us away from our own past and existing patterns and opens up fresh pathways of thinking.

ix) Volunteering for community work helps restore self-esteem and dilutes stress.

x) Creating a quiet, soothing corner of one's own. This could be decorated with cushions, lamps, scented candles, crystals, images of our favourite deities, loved ones, friends, our icons etc. along with attractive plants or an aquarium. Being in this space, whether to meditate or think or read, produces a sense of comfort and safety.

xii) Following a programme of regular exercise, whether alone or with partners, is a powerful mood elevator as it floods the body with endorphins and energy.

xiii) Letting go of unhealthy and toxic relationships.

xiv) Writing grudges on a piece of paper and then consigning the paper to the flames, thus releasing the grudges, one by one. This is a good way of aligning our mind with positivity. We can reward ourselves in whichever manner we deem fit as we let go of each grudge. This a powerful way of discarding negative thought patterns.

xv) Undergoing deep-tissue oil massage and acupressure therapies, which are excellent ways to release stress stored in the body.

Ayurveda and mental maladies

लोभशोकभयक्रोधमानवेगान् विधारयेत्‌।
नैर्लज्ज्येर्ष्यातिरागाणामभिध्यायाश्च बुद्धिमान्‌॥ २७॥—*Charaka Samhita*

*Lobhshokbhaykrodhmaanvegaan vidhyaryet
Nairlajyershatiragaraambhidhyayashch buddhiman.*

(A wise person should suppress mental urges pertaining to
the following:

lobha—greed, *shoka*—grief, *bhaya*—fear, *krodha*—anger,
mana—vanity, *nirlajja*—shamelessness, *irshya*—jealousy,
atiraga—excessive desire, *abhidhyaya*—malice)

Long before western medicine drew a connection between
mind and body, in the second century A.D., Acharya
Charaka, one of the founding fathers of Ayurveda, posited
that the origins of all diseases are in *manasa-vikara* or mental
afflictions. These afflictions of mind can be categorized thus:

1) *Kama* (lust): This refers to an intense and overwhelming
   desire for bodily pleasures. Lust can also include
   a craving for expressions of romantic love with or
   without sexual connotation. While kama or desire is an
   inevitable orientation among humans, it is important
   that the expression of kama is firmly rooted in a sense
   of awareness. Unbridled lust can act upon the brain like
   a drug. Overwhelming desire can generate obsessions

and feelings of anxiety. Such feelings can result in psychopathic behaviour and physical illness.

2) *Krodh* (anger): Anger is universally acknowledged as being one of the seven deadly sins of the human mind. This is because of its capacity to cause destruction. Anger aims at annihilating any opposition to one's egoistic choices. Expressions of anger vary from throwing hysterical tantrums to being verbally violent and a whole range of forms in between, including passive aggression. Apart from causing harm to those around, krodh can cause headaches, digestion issues, abdominal pain, heightened anxiety, depression, high blood pressure, skin problems like eczema, insomnia, heart attack and even paralytic stroke in an angry person.

3) *Shok* (grief): This emotion comes mainly from a loss of people or objects or situations dear to us. Along with uncontrolled grief comes aggravated vata and pitta dosha, leading to many ill effects. Grief can lead to forms of inflammation and batter the immune system, leaving us vulnerable to infection. When we are experiencing the condition of a 'broken heart', it is likely that our blood pressure shoots up, throwing our limbic system and the prefrontal cortex out of balance. This can affect our concentration levels and memory functions. A prolonged period of shok can, in extreme cases, cause one to fall terminally ill—which is rare, but possible.

4) *Bhay* (fear): Bhay occurs when we are confronted with an unwanted situation and are scared to the point of numbness. Sudden fear can precipitate both physical

and mental diseases. Our vata dosha is impacted, leading to bodily tremors, giddiness and dryness of mouth. Bhay can compromise our immune system and cause irreparable damage to the cardiovascular system. In the gastrointestinal system, fear can lead to ulcers and irritable bowel syndrome. Sustained or repeated bouts of fear can lead to swift ageing and in extreme situations, even premature death.

5) *Lobha* (greed): Gluttony can cause us to crave things in excess, whether it is wealth, attention, power, food or romantic love. It makes a person possessive and degrades their innate sense of nobility. A person afflicted by lobha may attempt to control others, leading to intense friction. Lobha for food will result in excess body fat, disrupted hunger regulation, excessive gas and bloating. Outwardly lobha manifests as selfishness, anger, jealousy and an unhealthy competitiveness.

6) *Matsarya* (jealousy): This stems from a sense of over-attachment or inferiority. It is also a part of 'passion-lust', which makes a person chronically possessive. It is invariably an incapacity to enjoy one's own possessions together with an inability to share. Jealousy manifests as futile comparisons and a tendency to cling. Jealousy triggers our body's stress responses and can lead to a whole range of stress-related disorders.

7) *Harsha* (excessive happiness): True happiness is a balanced and moderated mental state of well-being. It ranges from simple contentment to immense joy. However, sometimes, in pursuit of an extreme ecstatic

state, people tend to choose routes that are detrimental to health, such as certain extreme religious practices, addictions and substance abuse. While the method itself is often damaging to health, the outcome too can result in hysteria, euphoria and uncontrollable states of ecstasy. True happiness is produced by a balance of satva, rajas and tamoguna. Excessive harsha can, in extreme cases, lead to *hridayroga* (heart disease), delusion and even death.

8) *Madh* (arrogance): Arrogance can be defined as an excess of ego. Ego in itself is not a bad thing. According to Ayurveda, we are born out of cosmic selfishness or ahamkar, which is fundamental to our survival. However, arrogance is an excess of ahamkar. It is a common trait in pitta dominant people. It is a quality that can be inherited or it could be transmitted by our social and cultural environment. It is extremely damaging to the person's social relationships and their spiritual progress. It is a destructive quality that leads to isolation, depression, stress and illness.

Personality has implications for a person's health, career, social relationships and, in fact, every aspect of their life. Ayurveda offers a theoretical and empirical base of personality traits and types through an understanding of the play of gunas and doshas. This understanding makes it possible to offer holistic solutions for afflictions of the mind and consequently the body.

15

The Path of Meditation

Ayurveda is a science that explains the body in the context of the mind and beyond that, in the context of the cosmos. As humans, we have limited power over the mechanics of the body as these are pre-programmed. We have even less power over the immutable laws of the cosmos. The one area where we do have agency is that of the mind. They who have gained some level of mastery over the mind can influence the working of their body and even their environment. Meditation is the path to taking charge and taking responsibility for our own health and the health of our social and natural environment.

Meditation can be of many forms, but the objective of all of them is to calm the mind and stabilize the body. Meditation can take the form of mantra, prayers, dhyana, yoga, physical exercise and breathing practices.

Of these, dhyana is considered the most superior. It can be variously translated to mean profound contemplation or reflection and is the sixth limb of yoga. Dhyana helps the mind transcend the field of activity, leading to total relaxation of the body. It causes the metabolic rate to drop and the body to drastically reduce the production of stress hormones, such as cortisol and adrenaline. When we are in a deep meditative state, the body experiences a surge of serotonin, the chemical that regulates mood and creates a sense of well-being. When a person is ill, along with medication, Ayurveda prescribes meditation to help the body-mind mechanism repair itself organically.

Meditation is a tool to help us empty the countless unnecessary thoughts that clutter the mind. In 2005, the National Science Foundation in the US published an article that stated that, on an average, a person thinks anywhere between 12,000 to 60,000 thoughts a day.[17] We believe thoughts are good and that they guide us. That is, in fact, a fallacy. The study showed that 80 per cent of those thoughts were negatively oriented. That means that the mind is feeding the system a majority of thoughts that are dark, destructive and depressing. Moreover, about 75 per cent of the thoughts we had on the previous day are repeated. When my mother Madhu Sharma was recovering from cancer, she often told me that talking to oneself is beneficial. Positive self talk is a conscious decision to support one's mind and bodily functions. She had coined a prayer which she recited to herself several times a day; 'God is great . . . God is kind . . .

I'm in the pink of my health and all is well . . . I'm fit as a fiddle and all the happiness is mine.' She made a full recovery and all along, her BP was under control. When her doctor told her, 'Mrs Sharma, you're fit as a fiddle,' she knew her body has responded to the recitation. If we do not take charge of our thoughts, our habitual patterns are capable of causing immense harm to our health and well-being.

Hence, cleansing or emptying the mind regularly is an absolute necessity for a person to grow a healthy interior, which then reflects in the exterior. When we empty our mind of its thought content, our consciousness flows beyond the border of self-identity and attains an awareness of all-inclusiveness. Vasant Lad says, 'In that effortless state of awareness, you realize your true nature, which is peace and love and that state is supported in every cell by *para ojas*. In other words, para ojas opens the door to God consciousness, which is non-judgemental awareness. Then para ojas becomes soma, which releases molecules of bliss through the body.'[18]

Meditation is an active and dynamic engagement with our inner self to tap into the 'ultimate source' energy. Setting aside even 10 minutes every day for a meditation practice can fundamentally improve the quality of our lives. We are blessed that we have a vast selection of meditation practices to choose from, derived from many spiritual traditions: the Hindu *japa*/mantra meditation, the Buddhist Vipassana meditation, the Christian meditation based on scriptural verse contemplation and the Murāqabah Sufi meditation are all pathways to align ourselves with the universal creative energy and the creator.

Meditation as per your dosha

Walking meditation

When kapha is predominant, it will cause mental fogginess, which is not conducive to dhyana. In that case, a person needs movement to counter the heaviness of the mind. Walking meditation is a way of energizing and restoring clarity and focus. Walking with an awareness of mind is a great form of meditation that clears our mental cobwebs. One can walk outdoors or indoors. It is best to walk without shoes. Begin with three deep breaths before you start walking. Walking meditation is a Buddhist technique whereby it is recommended that as you walk, you watch your breath and fix your gaze on the ground. You may become aware of three stages of activity of your feet: planting the sole, sustaining the foot and then raising it off the ground. Doing this brings to your mind an acute sense of focus. Remind yourself to feel good about each cycle. In a while, one begins to feel happy and relaxed. Kapha-dominant people can choose any form of meditation that involves movement such as yoga, gardening or even house cleaning. What is important is that whatever form you choose, it must be done with mindfulness and inward awareness.

Breathing meditation

When pitta troubles you with its heat and edginess, you may feel irritated, frustrated or enraged. To cool yourself down, Ayurveda recommends forms of breathing meditation.

Pranayama is a field of yoga that relates to regulating the breath for physiological and emotional benefits. In Sanskrit, 'prana' means life energy and '*yama*' means control. The goal of pranayama is to synchronize your body and mind and it has immense health benefits. When pranayama is practised in conjunction with dhyana, it becomes a powerful tool of meditation.

Sit comfortably in a quiet, cool corner. Play some soothing music if you wish and release your thoughts as they arise. Consciously relax each muscle from the toes to the crown of your head. Then, in that relaxed state, simply begin observing your breath as it comes and goes. Do not attempt to control the breath, simply observe. After a while, you will be able control the frequency and duration of each breath. This is pranayama. As you observe the breath, it becomes the focus of your full attention. This is dhyana. Together, it is a form of breathing meditation that will calm the pitta nature, deliver huge physical and mental benefits and eventually, open the door to spiritual benefits. It is recommended to incorporate 15–20 minutes of this practice into your daily routine.

Mantra meditation

When there is a predominance of vata, a person feels unsettled, restless or anxious. In such cases, Ayurveda recommends mantra meditation as a tool to still the mind. The practice of mantra meditation utilizes the silent repetition of a word or a phrase as a point of focus to help slow mental activity and thought. The vibrations of certain Sanskrit words and phrases carry an energetic essence that support one's intentions. A mantra can be chosen in accordance with a person's own vibrations or one that supports their specific intention.

Just as instructed above, practice your mantra meditation in a quiet, happy space in the home. You may use beads if you wish. Close your eyes and begin by softly repeating your mantra. Visualize a white ball of light embracing you in its healing protection. In the initial days, you may chant aloud but as you progress, the chanting becomes an internalized, inward process that immerses you in its silent vibrations, to the exclusion of all outer disturbances or thought distractions.

Once you start living in such harmonious rhythms with your mind-body constitution, it will be easier for you to journey to the higher purposes of your life.

Meditation explained by Vasant Lad

Para and apara are the two types of ojas present within us. Para, the superior ojas, is located in the heart. Apara, the inferior ojas, circulates through the body.

According to Vasant Lad, 'Meditation is an effortless state where the mind becomes absolutely quiet and para ojas becomes active.'[19]

One form of meditation is to simply surrender to one's environment and remain in the present moment, without any interfering thoughts or judgements.

Self-Care

Taking care of ourselves should be our highest priority. This is something that is not always clearly understood. Most people consider it a luxury and something that we do in our free time. They could not be more mistaken. Because if we do not care for ourselves then nobody will. Self-care is also a mark of good mental health because it means we are psychologically self-reliant. We have taken responsibility and ownership of our life and are not mentally dependent on others for our well-being. Patriarchal cultures condition women not to prioritize themselves. Instead, they are raised to be caregivers. This leads to immense physical and psychological damage to traditionally raised women.

It is important to assess whether we are taking care of ourselves. Do we have a constructive and useful attitude to address and process our emotions? Are we practically incorporating those practices into our daily life? Are we putting our stress triggers into perspective so that they do not overwhelm us? Are we living with full awareness and mindfulness?

Strange though it may sound, most people sleepwalk through life. Living a mindful life and being conscious of how precious the gift of life is is the key to mental health. Even if our circumstances are not always fair or perfect, mindful living enables us to recognize our triggers and address them in a calm, constructive manner. Self-help is the path to self-empowerment.

Each of us needs to design a self-help schedule for ourselves. There is no 'one size' that fits all and we need to create schedules, practices and methods that work best for us.

Creative visualization

This method has been found to be greatly effective in offering us a metaphysical route to the kind of life we deeply wish for and deserve to live. This is achieved by guiding our imagination on a daily basis to feel that we are in a happy space. We visualize ourselves as having an abundance of love and resources. In this way, it becomes possible to positively rewrite the impressions of our brain's neural pathways. Since mind and cosmos are interconnected, positive visualization techniques have the potential to bring about real changes in our circumstances.

As an example of creative visualization:

> I focus on my breath and practice conscious breathing by breathing in positivity and breathing out love. I also breathe out negative thoughts like hatred and jealousy. Further, while focusing on my breath, I breathe in a feeling of wellness for myself and breathe out a feeling of wellness for others.

Positive affirmation

Positive affirmation involves positive self-talk with gratitude. It works in the same manner as a mantra except that it holds specific meaning for the person and resonates with their wishes. We need to formulate the mantra/affirmation best suited to us. A daily repetition causes the positive thought or feeling to remain in the mind through the day.

Studies have shown that positive affirmations yield impressive results. Some examples are:

(i)   I am happy, I am healthy, I feel terrific.
(ii)   I am happy with my solitude.
(iii) I love and accept myself.
(iv)   My heart keeps me safe.
(v)   I am sustained by the love of God.
(vi)   I always make right choices.
(vii) I will do whatever is good for me.
(viii) Today will be a happy day for me.
(ix)   I forgive all and I am free.
(x)   I am appreciated and rewarded for my work.
(xi)   My family loves me more every day.
(xii) I choose friends who are my emotional support in a positive way.

The power of love

There are few substitutes for love. Indeed, it is the fundamental need of all sentient beings. We should endeavour to cultivate loving relationships around us, whether with our partners, parents, children, friends or pets. Without at least a few loving relationships in one's life, a person can become depressed, violent and isolated. Physical proximity with a loved one is a tonic to the mind and body.

However, even without other people, it is possible to experience a self-generated feeling of unconditional, all-encompassing, boundless, ineffable love. This is because a loving union is the very nature of the universal consciousness. In moments of deep meditation, it is possible for the practitioner to be transformed by a foretaste of this divine love.

'To love oneself is the beginning of a life-long romance.'— Oscar Wilde

'To fall in love with yourself is the secret to happiness.'— Robert Morley

Aromatherapy

Recent research has proved that certain aromas can alter the activity of the brain waves and lower stress hormones. Therefore, lighting scented candles, keeping potpourri sachets and fresh flowers or using scented bath oils/salts and perfumes are recommended as wonderful self-help practices. Fragrances arouse our sense of refinement and make us feel loved and pampered.

Hobbies

It is important to indulge ourselves by doing things that we enjoy. Paint, sing, dance or do whatever it is that makes you happy. Such activities allow us to express and release emotions. It is interesting to note that there is a worldwide demand for adult colouring books. Hitherto considered a children's activity, colouring books have now been found to be deeply therapeutic for adults as well.

Prayer

Prayer and even religious rituals are powerful tools for soothing and strengthening ourselves and maintaining our mental equilibrium. When everything fails, it is our faith that keeps us going. It is imperative that we care for our spiritual health. Research shows that prayer delivers benefits similar to meditation—it can calm the nervous system and shut down the fight-or-flight response. It can make a person less reactive to negative emotions and reduce stress. Research also demonstrates that patients who have a strong faith have a higher tolerance for pain and are more likely to recover from life-threatening illnesses. 'A 2004 study on religious coping methods in the *Journal of Health Psychology* found that people who approach God as a partner or a collaborator in their lives had better mental and physical health outcomes.'[20]

16

The Ancient Roots of Ayurveda

The beginnings of Ayurveda are recorded in our ancient scriptures. The story of Ayurveda relates to the great cosmic churning, the Samudra Manthan, an event mentioned in ancient texts such as the *Bhagavata Purana,* the Mahabharata and the *Vishnu Purana.*

The story goes that once upon a time, Indra, king of the *devas*, mounted on his elephant, happened to pass the home of the sage Durvasa. Stepping out of his modest dwelling in the forest, Durvasa offered Indra a wreath of flowers. Indra accepted the flowers carelessly and tossed it onto his elephant's trunk. The strong fragrance of the flowers irritated the elephant and it threw the wreath onto the ground, trampling it into the dust. It is never wise to anger a sage, even if you are king of the gods, and Durvasa was furious at the disrespect shown to him. He cursed Indra, saying that henceforth, the devas would no longer be immortal.

When the devas in the heavens lost their power, the *asuras*, who ruled the netherworld, began to rise up against them. So the devas rushed to Vishnu, the preserver of the universe, in a panic and begged him to restore their immortality. Vishnu advised them to make peace with the asuras and to join forces with them to procure *amrit*, the elixir of immortality, and the many other treasures that lay deep under the ocean. The asuras were told that if they cooperated, the gifts of the ocean would be shared equally. But Vishnu secretly promised the devas that only they would receive the amrit, restoring their dominance over the asuras.

The devas and asuras came together to churn the ocean to bring forth the amrit. Using the Mandara mountain as a churning rod and Vasuki the celestial snake as the rope, the devas and asuras began churning the celestial waters. To prevent Mount Mandara from sinking to the bottom of the ocean, Vishnu took the form of a turtle, the *kurma* avatar, and dove into the ocean, supporting the mountain on his back. And thus were the waters of *samsara* churned to yield its treasures.

Many mystical creatures and objects rose to the surface until Dhanvantari finally emerged, the divine physician and the fount of Ayurveda. In popular iconography, Dhanvantri is depicted as a glowing youth dressed in yellow silk. Around his neck he wears a necklace of tulsi seeds and on his head, a wreath made of medicinal herbs. In his four hands he bears a chakra, a golden leech for bloodletting, the *Upaveda*, the source of the science of Ayurveda, and finally, a pot containing the elixir of immortality.

The story of the Samudra Manthan is well known. While there are many interpretations, Ayurveda practitioners explain it thus: Ayurveda sees life and health as emerging from dynamic balance, and that dynamic balance is conveyed here through the analogy of the churning of the ocean. Ayurveda teaches that the properties associated with an element or mahabhuta emerge only in a state of activation. For instance, if a substance produces heaviness in the body, then it is understood that the earth element (prithvi mahabhuta) is present in it in an activated state. The activation of the elements in the body takes place through *a churning*. In other words, if the five elements are what constitute reality, it is *samudra manthan* that activates their qualities. The churning within the human mind-body complex takes place between the two poles of our inner devas and asuras, who represent the elements of akash (ether) and prithvi (earth), where prithvi is our material or base nature and akash our divine nature. Between these two poles lie the remaining three elements of water, fire and air, which are mapped into the doshas of vata, pitta and kapha. The churning has the potential to create balance or imbalance. It is only when it is supported by dharma, or right living and right thinking, symbolized by Vishnu in the form of a turtle, that we can experience true health.

In the story, Dhanvantri presents himself to Lord Vishnu and, bowing to him, says, 'Oh Lord, I am your son. Allot a share of the celestial gifts to me.' But Vishnu refuses. He says, 'Portions have already been allotted. Since you were born after the celestials, you cannot be considered as one of

medical treatise of his own, there is a voluminous glossary and materia medica known as *Dhanvantari Niganthu.*

Dhanvantari's disciples also took on the honorific title of Dhanvantri, indicative of their proficiency in the science. Even today, the title is used by master vaids. Dhanvantri is worshipped today as the patron deity and protector of Ayurveda practitioners. While there are temples dedicated to Dhanvantri all over India, the more prominent ones are in the southern states of Kerala and Tamil Nadu. He is worshipped with a mantra that roughly translates to:

'We pray to the God Dhanvantri, he who holds the pot with the nectar of immortality. Lord Dhavantri eliminates all fears and diseases, because he is merciful, he is the guardian of the three worlds, beloved of Vishnu, healer of the soul. We honour him.'

Another one invokes him thus:

'Greetings to Dhanvantri, who holds in his four hands a shell, herbs, leeches and amrita. In whose heart shines the purest, most delicate, blessed light. This light shines around his head and around his lotus eyes. He who, with only one look, destroys all illnesses like a huge forest fire.'

In the northern states, Dhanvantri is worshipped along with the goddess Lakshmi on the festival of Dhanteras two days ahead of Diwali.

There is another myth that states that the original teaching of the sacred science of life (Ayurveda) was first offered in the mysterious realm of the gods, when Brahma, the creator of the universe, gave it to Daksha, his son, who was born out of Brahma's right thumb. Daksha transmitted the knowledge of Ayurveda to two heavenly beings called the Ashwini twins—heavenly healers—who then gave it to Indra, king of the heavens. Indra revealed it to the people of the earth through the great sage and maharishi Bhardvaja, who then imparted the knowledge to Atreya, a spiritually perfected being. The teachings of Atreya were edited and codified by his disciple Charaka in what is arguably the most ancient medical book in the world, the *Charaka Samhita*. This and the *Sushruta Samhita* are the two foundational Ayurveda texts that have survived from 100 B.C.

In the Hindu culture, the lines between history and myth, matter and spirit, blur easily and constantly. Therefore, it is appropriate that the science of Ayurveda aims at healing not only the body but also the soul. It aims to rebalance the energies in the body to repair the connection between the body and the higher self, and in so doing, restore the balance and harmony between the human and society, between the human and the environment and between the human and the cosmos, of which the human is a microcosm.

17

The Spiritual Blessings of Ayurveda

Spirituality is a concept broad and wide enough to hold many different perspectives on the same truth within the parameters of a cosmic ethic. The spiritual dimension of Ayurveda guides our physiology to connect us with something bigger and beyond the physical.

Ayurveda as a science helps to prepare our physical body for the journey into the knowledge of consciousness itself. In its schemata, a healthy physical body is a device for attaining self-knowledge. Thus, Ayurveda's magnificent physio-spiritual perspective teaches us that we are 'spirit' in essence but undergoing a human or a bodily experience that is designed to evolve us into a union with the highest truth, that is God. On our way to this greatest destination, whatever health challenges our body faces can be healed by using natural herbs, minerals, metals and other bounties of

Mother Earth. Ayurveda heals us so that we get to use our lives for our ultimate purpose: self-realization.

From darkness to light—this journey is illustrated by the Ayurvedic concept of the three gunas: tamas, rajas and satva. All three are inevitable states through which our mind and consequently, our body, pass. Tamas, as we know by now, is the state of darkness. It represents a state of our psyche that has no knowledge of its own source. Who am I? Where did I come from? To where am I proceeding? In the state of tamas, we remain deprived of knowledge about ourselves. This ignorance causes us to fall into *moha* or desires for repetitive experiences through our body-mind identity, in which we act selfishly, believing we are alone and we must defend and protect our interest above anyone else's. Tamas or the darkness of ignorance causes us to even resort to violence, narrow-mindedness, prejudices or inertia. We remain trapped in a cycle of fear, guilt and addictions.

As we progress on the spiritual path, other frequencies and vibrations stir within us. What Ayurveda refers to as rajas puts us in a state of action and activities that motivate us to create a world of our liking and desires. We then progress into intensely challenging material experiences of conquests and thrills, anxieties and attachments and consequently, disappointments. Finally, when we move to the state of satva within us, we attain a totally different level of perception. Our vision turns deeper, clearer and purer. We start seeing the connection between parts and pieces that appear separated in the cosmos. We ask the deeper questions. We ask who we are and from whence we came and we start receiving the answers.

Each individual knows that he or she will not remain in a body beyond a certain span of time. And thus, in a state of satva, men and women ask themselves as they grow serene in mind: 'If this earth and this body of mine were my real home, where I belong, then why am I forced to leave it?' In the state of satva, we thus awaken and seek conscious reality.

The divine meaning of life

Ayurveda empowers us in this journey by keeping us closest to our true nature and giving us the gift of a healthy body as a device for this enquiry. That is precisely why Ayurveda does not encourage us to take medicine mindlessly. Instead, it shows us our bodily truths. Then it tames our nature and steers us to a faith in the divine meaning of life. Of course, Ayurvedic potions would work on any man or woman, believer or not. But when accepted through faith in one's own true dharma, Ayurvedic medicines are capable of working wonders in us. Whenever medicine is taken, it is best taken in total faith. For when we raise our faith to a point where it is larger than our fears, we are gifted a life that is peaceful. Our faith in our ethics, our well-being and in our dharma will enhance our spiritual capabilities, and before long, our fears will vanish. And that is the key to living well. Faith nourishes our ojas, tejas and prana as well. When we develop the habit of faith, our mind becomes conditioned to healing and health.

Ayurveda teaches us that the path to holistic healing is through self-knowledge and self-empowerment. This healing system not only addresses our physical bodies but our mental and spiritual aspects too, for in truth, there is no separation between the three. The Roman philosopher Cicero's famous dictum states: 'Diseases of the soul are both more dangerous and more numerous than those of the body.'[21]

The body as a holy shrine

'A well-lived day is medicine unto itself.'—Acharya Shunya

We have already examined the role of food in keeping us in good health. Besides food, our thoughts, speech and actions also play important roles in our well-being. Ayurveda encourages us to look upon our physical being as a temple and to revere it. How do we revere a place of worship? By accepting its sacred nature and keeping it clean and protected. To consecrate our body into a sacred structure, we offer it only foods and beverages that nourish it and not those that would harm it. Who would throw junk into a sacred space? It is natural for sattvic eating habits to grow out of this understanding of our body as a temple. In turn, once the body is nourished by good nutrients, cleansing food, right exercise and meditation etc., it will replenish itself with a fresh supply of ojas and tejas. This eventually leads to *vivek*— intellect or clear discernment. You then proceed through life with clarity about what is moral and to be accepted, and what is immoral and to be rejected. Whenever we think, speak and act without clear discernment, we lose contact with our inner awareness and consciousness. This leads us to think, speak and act out of vested interests, which may harm our fellow beings and even our own body and mind. Such a wrongful way of living will eventually lead to diseases. Ayurveda calls this *pragyaparadh*—mistake of the intellect. Whether we are consciously spiritual or not, when we act out of an awareness of the connectedness of all beings, we will be led by the eternal light of consciousness. Physical well-being begins in your inner space, on the level of the mind, before it manifests physically. As Swami Vivekananda taught, 'You have to grow from the inside out. None can teach you, none can make you spiritual. There is no other teacher but your own soul.'[22]

Dharma shows you the path

As humans, we are bound to do some karma. There are two ways of approaching karma: selfless karma and desired karma. In the first instance, you do whatever comes your way, doing what needs to be done without any concern about the results. The second is born out of your desire to do. You may engage in such karma if you are watchful of the morals of the results. Is it harmful to any being in this cosmos? Is my selfishness alone my motivation here? Am I unsettling the harmony of the larger whole? It is important to weigh all these questions before proceeding. Accepting spiritual responsibilities in life situations results in having a strong moral and ethical foundation for the edifice of your life. This keeps you stable and balanced. Your mind stays stable and aligns with an awareness of quotidian ethics. This alignment with dharma helps your life flow peacefully.

Dharma involves being truthful, practising non-violence, having good morals and being aware of the workings of karma. If we incorporate dharma into Ayurveda, it makes us mindful of the immutable laws of karma. If you hurt the cosmos, the hurt comes right back at you because you are not separate from your cosmos. And that robs you of your own peace. If you are not at peace, you cannot be in good health either. Guilt, anxieties, worries, doubts, fears etc. ruin a person's physical and mental stability. The path of Ayurveda shows us how to find health through living in harmony with our own conscience—a state of being that is worth more than anything else in life. Ayurveda encourages you to take refuge in the principles of spirituality.

May the holy path of Ayurveda bless you with a life of serendipity and transcendence! May the gurus of this sacred science guide your every step! May the ultimate healer bless you with good health!

Om shanti, shanti, shanti . . .

Shiv Shankar
Lord of creation,
Light of light
Supreme consciousness of which we are all a part.
Adi deva—first among the gods
Mahadev—highest among the gods
Adiyogi—preceptor of yoga
Guru of all gurus.

Shiv Shakti
You are the only reality, the sum of all that is
All-pervading, omniscient, omnipresent, omnipotent.
You are the thought behind every action, the action itself and
the outcome.
You are the chants and the worship,
You are the ritual and the recipient of the ritual.
Every prayer, to every god, is a prayer to you.
You are in all beauty and in all brilliance,
You are love itself,
You are ever merciful,
Your glories are infinite and unparalleled.
A million salutations, o supreme one!

(Prayer adapted from the teachings of 'Mother', Vedanta Guru)

Notes

1. Ex-director of Institute for Ayurvedic Research & Studies, Jamnagar and of the Bandarnaike Memorial Ayurvedic Research Institute, Navinna, Ceylon as well as advisor on Ayurveda to the Government of Ceylon.

2. Padma Bhushan and Padma Vibhushan and an authority on Nadi Vaidyam or pulse diagnosis.

3. Konstantin G. Korotkov, 'Study of structured water and its biological effects', *International Journal of Complementary & Alternative Medicine*, 7 October 2019, https://www.researchgate. net/publication/342162300_Study_of_structured_water_and_ its_biological_effects/.

4. Sadhguru, 'The Science of Theerth, Isha Foundation, 29 July 2019, https://isha.sadhguru.org/in/en/wisdom/article/spiritual- significance-water-india.

5. Lauren Gernady, 'Which Direction Do You Sleep In? According to Ayurveda, It Matters', Kripalu Center for Yoga & Health, https://kripalu.org/resources/which-direction-do-you-sleep- according-ayurveda-it-matters.

6. Alain Danielou, tr., *The Complete Kama Sutra*, (Rochester: Vermont: Inner Traditions, 1993).

7. 'Understanding sexual energy- spiritually', The Dancing Yogi, 22 January 2022, https://trinketsofexistence2.wordpress.com/2022/01/22/understanding-sexual-energy-spiritually/.

8. *Sharirasthana*, II.38-44.

9. *Chikitsasthana*, XXX.34.

10. Sutra 2.38.

11. Sri Swami Sivananda, 'Brahmacharya (Celibacy)', The Divine Life Society, https://www.dlshq.org/teachings/brahmacharya-celibacy/.

12. Arpita Mitra, 'Concentration: An Important Component in Swami Vivekananda's Idea of Education', Vivekananda International Foundation, 11 January 2021, https://www.vifindia.org/2021/january/11/concentration-an-important-component-in-swami-vivekananda-s-idea-of-education.

13. The Mystic World, 'ASTONISHING POWERS! See What Happens When You Practice This', YouTube, 1 August 2022, https://www.youtube.com/watch?v=TWG5P_dQvew/.

14. Vasant Lal, *Textbook of Ayurveda: Fundamental Principles* (Ayurvedic Press, 2002), vol. 1, p. 133.

15. 'Fasting for Health and Longevity: Nobel Prize Winning Research on Cell Aging', Blue Zones, https://www.bluezones.com/2018/10/fasting-for-health-and-longevity-nobel-prize-winning-research-on-cell-aging/.

16. Enid Nemy, 'Frances Lear, a Mercurial Figure of the Media and a Magazine Founder, Dead at 73', *New York Times*, 1 October 1996, available at https://www.nytimes.com/1996/10/01/us/frances-lear-a-mercurial-figure-of-themedia-and-a-magazine-founder-dead-at-73.html.

17. Neringa Antanaityte, 'Mind Matter: How To Effortlessly Have More Positive Thoughts', TLEX Institute, https://tlexinstitute.com/how-to-effortlesslyhave-more-positive-thoughts/.

18. Vasant Lal, *Textbook of Ayurveda: Fundamental Principles* (Ayurvedic Press, 2002), vol. 1, p. 212.

19. Vasant Lal, *Textbook of Ayurveda: Fundamental Principles* (Ayurvedic Press, 2002), vol. 1, p. 212.

20. Elizabeth Bernstein, 'The Science of Prayer', *Wall Street Journal*, 17 May 2020.

21. Cicero, *Tusculanae Disputationes*, book 3, chapter 3.

22. '10 quotes by Swami Vivekanand that continue to inspire us even today!', *Times of India*, 12 January 2021, https://timesofindia.indiatimes.com/life-style/books/features/quotes-by-swami-vivekananda-which-are-relevant-even-today/photostory/70072054.cms/.

Scan QR code to access the
Penguin Random House India website